Practical Clinical Research Design and Application

Peter D. Fabricant

Practical Clinical Research Design and Application

A Primer for Physicians, Surgeons, and Clinical Healthcare Professionals

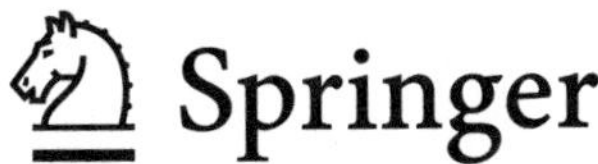 Springer

Peter D. Fabricant, MD, MPH
Associate Professor of Orthopedic Surgery
Hospital for Special Surgery
New York, NY, USA

ISBN 978-3-031-58382-7   ISBN 978-3-031-58380-3   (eBook)
https://doi.org/10.1007/978-3-031-58380-3

This Springer imprint is published by the registered company Springer Nature Switzerland AG
The registered company address is: Gewerbestrasse 11, 6330 Cham, Switzerland

If disposing of this product, please recycle the paper

Preface

The practice of medicine and surgery requires dedication to lifelong learning. As such, every practicing physician, surgeon, advanced practice provider, and allied health professional interacts regularly with peer-reviewed literature, either while creating it or consuming it. Despite the countless hours over many years spent in formal clinical training, many clinicians and clinician-authors lack advanced training or a working nuanced knowledge of research methodology and study design. Institutions have responded to this gap by reinforcing their ranks with statistical and methodological support in the form of data analysts, epidemiologists, and biostatisticians. However, clinicians are too often unable to "talk the methodological talk" to guide them. This ultimately results in a stark disconnect between clinically relevant aspects of research (i.e., what clinicians want to study) and appropriate study design (i.e., choosing and executing the correct methodology to answer the question).

I wrote this book after realizing the need for a concise, readable, and practical guide for clinicians to read and reference. Although many textbooks will "get into the weeds" with statistical and epidemiological theory and equations, they are not easily digestible by trainees and practicing clinicians who want pragmatic knowledge of this content in order to design their own studies or enhance their understanding of the medical literature.

It is my hope that this book can serve as a standalone text "written by a clinician, for clinicians," but from the perspective of someone with formal training in research methodology, biostatistics, and epidemiology.

New York, NY, USA

Peter D. Fabricant, MD, MPH

Acknowledgments

I would like to sincerely thank Dr. Shevaun Doyle who inspired the idea for this book and spent many hours reviewing and editing the work, and Dr. Rob Rozbruch for helping formulate my ideas into a formal book proposal.

My wife, Dr. Son McLaren, deserves special recognition for her thoughtful and thorough editorial critique as well as serving as a friendly debate partner for much of this book's contents.

I would also like to thank my research assistants during this time, Preston Gross and Ruthie Jones, for their help with manuscript preparation and figure production.

Finally, I would like to acknowledge my mentors, colleagues, and Hospital for Special Surgery, all of whom have created an environment in which to build a thriving clinical practice while meaningfully contributing to research and education.

Contents

About the Author

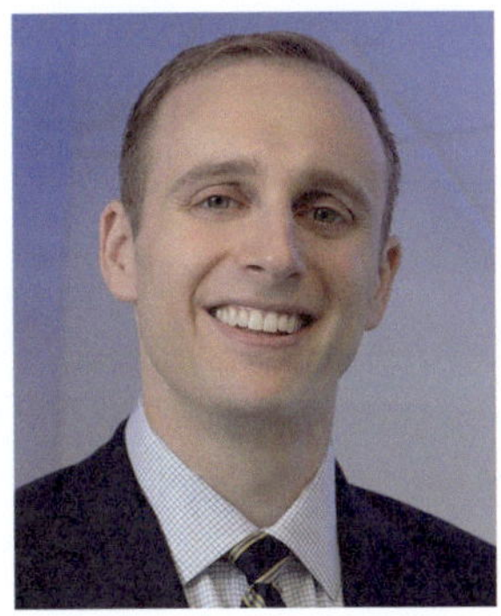

Peter D. Fabricant, MD, MPH is an attending orthopedic surgeon on the Pediatric Orthopedic Surgery Service at Hospital for Special Surgery (HSS) and Associate Professor of Orthopedic Surgery at Weill Cornell Medical College in New York, NY. He holds a dual appointment in the Research Division at HSS and serves as the Education Director for the Pediatric Orthopedic Surgery Service and Associate Residency Program Director. He is a clinician-scientist specializing in pediatric and adolescent sports injuries, trauma, clinical outcomes, and quality improvement research.

Dr. Fabricant completed his undergraduate studies with honors at the University of Rochester, and then attended Yale University School of Medicine. During his orthopedic surgery residency training at HSS, he earned a Master of Public Health degree from Columbia University Mailman School of Public Health.

Dr. Fabricant has an extensive publication and speaking record in pediatric and adolescent orthopedic surgery, sports medicine, and trauma. He has developed a reputation as a clinical and research mentor to medical students and orthopedic surgery residents and fellows, and spends considerable time lecturing and consulting on clinical research and study design locally, regionally, and internationally.

Dr. Fabricant's recent investigations have spanned several areas including clinical outcomes, quality improvement, cost-effectiveness, health policy and economics, outcome metrics and their psychometric properties, basic science, anatomy, and biomechanics. He lives in New York City with his wife, Dr. Son McLaren, their daughter, Avery, and their cat, Bruin.

Part I
Foundational Basics

Chapter 1
Descriptive Statistics

Introduction

Descriptive statistics provide researchers with a set of techniques to summarize and describe the main features of a dataset. They allow researchers to systematically organize, analyze, and concisely interpret numerical data. Researchers are then able to distill complex information into meaningful and manageable summaries to identify patterns, detect outliers, and make informed decisions on how to further analyze and interpret data. By understanding the nature of a dataset, researchers can refine hypotheses that may be investigated in greater depth using comparative statistics (described in Chaps. 2 and 3).

Types of Descriptive Statistics

Measures of Central Tendency

Univariable measures of central tendency describe the point estimate or center of a dataset. Examples include:

(a) **Mean**: The mean is the arithmetic average of a set of values. Means are used to describe the central tendency of normally distributed data (explained below), as they can be affected by outliers. For example, if there is a tight grouping of numbers but a single outlier is three times larger than the second highest value, this will skew the mean higher than would be a true measure of central tendency of the data. By "averaging in" the outlier, the mean is elevated higher than would have been the case without the outlier. This is even more problematic with smaller datasets where one or a few outliers can substantially skew the mean value of the data.

P. D. Fabricant, *Practical Clinical Research Design and Application*, https://doi.org/10.1007/978-3-031-58380-3_1

(b) **Median**: The median is the middle value that separates the upper and lower half of the data when arranged in increasing order. The median is also referred to as the 50th percentile. Medians can be used to describe the central tendency of both normally distributed (i.e., parametric) and non-normally distributed (i.e., non-parametric) data. They are not affected by outliers. Using the same example above, if there is a tight grouping of numbers but a single outlier is three times larger than the second highest value, this will not affect the median because the median value is the middle value of the ranked items.

(c) **Mode:** The mode is the value or values that appear most frequently in the dataset. It is not commonly used in clinical research and is usually only appropriate when describing nominal data (e.g., survey responses) rather than continuous data.

Measures of Variability

Measures of variability further describe a dataset by quantifying the spread or dispersion of the data around the measure of central tendency. Examples include:

(a) **Range**: Range is the difference between the maximum and minimum values in the dataset. This is substantially affected by outliers, as outliers tend to be the minimum or maximum values of a dataset and, therefore, are the values used to calculate the range.

(b) **Variance**: Variance is the mean squared deviation from the mean. To calculate variance, one would first calculate the mean, then find each data point's difference from the mean. Then, each of these values would be squared, and the sum of those squared values would be divided by one less than the sample size (n-1).

(c) **Standard Deviation**: Standard deviation is the square root of the variance, representing the average distance between each data point and the mean. Standard deviation is most commonly used as the measure of variability around a mean (e.g., with normally distributed data). This can be visually represented using a bar graph with error bars (Fig. 1.1).

(d) **Interquartile Range** (IQR): IQR is defined as the range between the first quartile (25th percentile) and third quartile (75th percentile) of the data. IQR is most commonly used as the measure of variability around a median (e.g., with non-normally distributed data). These non-parametric data are visually represented using a boxplot (Fig. 1.2).

(e) **Percentiles**: Percentiles divide the data into hundredths and describe the relative position of a value within the dataset. As mentioned above, the 50th percentile is equal to the median.

Fig. 1.1 Bar graph. A bar graph depicts normally distributed (parametric) continuous data. In this example, the bar heights represent the group means, and the error bars extend one standard deviation above and below the means. Bar graphs can also measure frequency (count) of categorical data but would not typically have error bars unless representing proportions

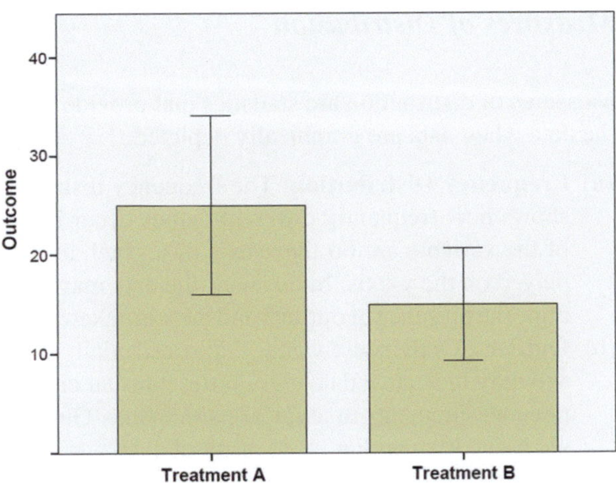

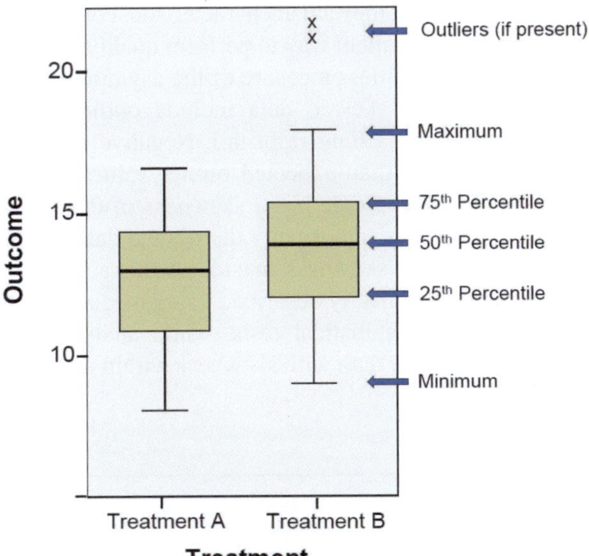

Fig. 1.2 Boxplot. A boxplot is a non-parametric graphical depiction of numerical data through their quartiles. The typical plot includes both a "box" and "whiskers." As noted in the figure, the box is defined by the 75th percentile at its upper limit, the 25th percentile at its lower limit, and an additional horizontal line denotes the median (or 50th percentile). The whiskers extending above and below represent the maximum and minimum data values, respectively, and must end at an observed data point. Whiskers may be portrayed in one of two ways: either as the true maximum and minimum (including any outliers), or using the 1.5 interquartile range (IQR) rule (as illustrated in the above figure). In the 1.5 IQR rule, whiskers are drawn from the upper and lower quartile a distance of 1.5 times the IQR to the furthest observed data point in that range. Additional outlier data are drawn individually

Measures of Distribution

Measures of distribution are statistics that provide information about the "shape" of the data when data are graphically depicted:

(a) **Frequency Distribution**: The frequency distribution is a table or a graph that shows how frequently different values occur in a dataset. Typically, the values of the variable are on the x-axis of a graph and the count or frequency is displayed on the y-axis. In this way, the data may be depicted graphically to determine the presence of outliers and measure skewness and kurtosis (defined below).

(b) **Outliers**: Outliers are values that substantially differ from the rest of the dataset and may indicate a data entry error, unusual or erroneous observations, or accurate measurements in atypical participants. Outliers are managed on an individual basis. If an outlier is the result of a data recording error, then those errors are corrected. If it is a result of an accurate measurement in an atypical participant, then those individuals are reconsidered for inclusion into or exclusion from the study based on the reason that they are uncharacteristic. For these reasons, screening for outliers can be an excellent way to perform quality control on a dataset.

(c) **Skewness**: Skewness is a unitless measure of the asymmetry of the data distribution. Positive or "right" skewed data include outliers with higher-than-expected outlier values and a long right tail. Negative or "left" skewed data include outliers with lower-than-expected outlier values and a long left tail. Perfectly normally distributed data has a skewness of 0; however, commonly accepted values for skewness of normally distributed data are between -2 and $+2$ [1] (Fig. 1.3). Data with skewness outside of this accepted range for normally distributed data are typically described using median and IQR and evaluated using non-parametric statistical tests, while analysis using parametric statistical tests is reserved for data with skewness within this accepted range for normally distributed data.

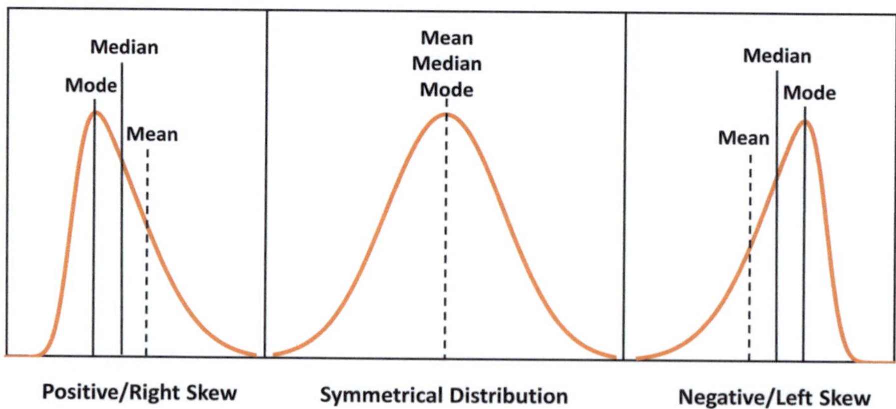

Fig. 1.3 Skewness

(d) **Kurtosis**: Kurtosis is a unitless measure of the peakedness or flatness of the data distribution. Compared to data that are normally distributed, data with positive kurtosis has a peaked curve and long tails, while data with negative kurtosis has a flatter curve and shorter tails. Perfectly normally distributed data exhibit a kurtosis of 0; however, commonly accepted values for kurtosis of normally distributed data are between -2 and $+2$ [1] (Fig. 1.4).

A symmetric distribution is depicted in the center panel (Fig. 1.3). In symmetrical distributions, the mean = median = mode. Positive or "right" skewed data (left panel) include outliers with higher-than-expected outlier values and a long right tail. In positive skewed data, the mean is greater than the median, which is greater than the mode. The skewed outliers affect the mean more than the median as these are "averaged in" to the dataset. Conversely, negative or "left" skewed data (right panel) include outliers with lower-than-expected outlier values and a long left tail. In negative skewed data, the mean is less than the median, which is less than the mode, because of the low value outliers "pulling down" the mean through averaging. Because skewed datasets affect the mean more than the median, data with skewness outside of the accepted range for normally distributed data (-2 to $+2$) are typically described using median and IQR, and evaluated using non-parametric statistical tests (Chaps. 2 and 3). Conversely, describing data using means and standard deviation and analysis using parametric statistical tests (Chaps. 2 and 3) are reserved for data with skewness within the accepted range for normally distributed data.

Normally distributed data are shown in orange (Fig. 1.4). Data with positive kurtosis exhibit a peaked curve and longer tails (green), while data with negative kurtosis demonstrate a flatter curve and shorter or nonexistent tails (blue).

Fig. 1.4 Kurtosis

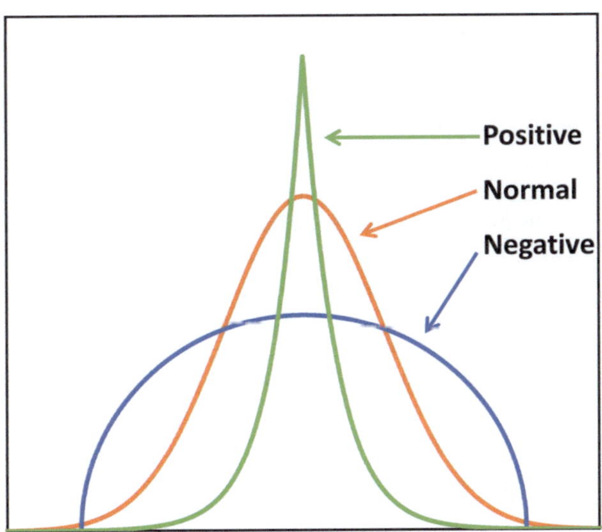

Importance of Descriptive Statistics

Tabulating and reporting the descriptive statistics of a dataset is a crucial first step in understanding the data and how to best further analyze it. Additionally, descriptive statistics provide a standard process with which to convey data to a reader in simple, straightforward terms. By providing a comprehensive overview of a dataset, descriptive statistics enable researchers, analysts, and decision-makers to understand its key characteristics, identify patterns, detect anomalies, and make informed decisions based on the data.

Six important roles of descriptive statistics include:

1. **Data Summarization**: Descriptive statistics allow us to condense large datasets into concise and meaningful summaries. By calculating measures of central tendency such as the mean, we can determine the typical or average value of a reported variable. These summary statistics provide a quick snapshot of the data, easing comprehension and communication of the information.
2. **Variability Assessment**: Descriptive statistics help us understand the variability or distribution of data within a dataset. Measures such as the range, variance, and standard deviation provide insights into how spread out the data points are from the central tendency. This knowledge is crucial for assessing the consistency, stability, and reliability of data, as well as in identifying outliers.
3. **Data Comparison**: Descriptive statistics are instrumental when it comes to comparing different datasets. By initially analyzing summary statistics, researchers are able to identify trends across various groups, populations, or timepoints. These comparisons allow the investigator to identify patterns, understand relationships, and determine factors that may influence the variables being investigated.
4. **Data Quality Assessment**: Descriptive statistics play a critical role in assessing data quality. By examining datasets for outliers, researchers can identify anomalous data points that may indicate errors, data entry mistakes, or aberrant observations. This ensures the integrity of the eventual analyses and minimizes the risk of drawing inaccurate or misleading conclusions.
5. **Communication and Visualization**: Descriptive statistics offer simple, quick, and effective ways to communicate data. Graphical depictions such as histograms, box plots, and scatter plots provide visual representations of data distributions, patterns, and relationships.
6. **Hypothesis Testing and Inference**: Descriptive statistics provide a solid foundation for further statistical analysis, including hypothesis testing and inferential statistics. By understanding the distribution and characteristics of the data through descriptive statistics, researchers can make informed decisions about appropriate further comparative statistical analyses.

Conclusion

In summary, descriptive statistics are used to summarize and describe the main features of a dataset. This way researchers can understand dataset characteristics, identify patterns, detect anomalies, generate hypotheses to test, and strategically perform more in depth comparative statistical analyses as described in Chaps. 2 and 3.

Reference

1. George D, Mallery P. IBM SPSS statistics 23 step by step: a simple guide and reference. 14th ed. New York, NY: Routledge; 2016. https://doi.org/10.4324/9781315545899.

Chapter 2
Comparative Statistics: Categorical Data

Introduction

Many measurements and clinical research outcomes are categorical. Although less granular or precise than continuous data (Chap. 3), categorical data structure is much easier to understand and is motivated by real-world concepts. Such real-world concepts include successful versus failed treatment, and good versus fair versus poor outcomes.

This chapter will review concepts around reporting and analyzing categorical data, including bivariable analyses (e.g., two-proportion z-tests and chi-squared tests) and multivariable analyses (e.g., logistic regression). Although the formulas for calculating test statistics are beyond the scope of this book, this chapter will provide insight into the concepts of categorical data analysis and the basic structure of a multiple logistic regression formula.

What Is Categorical Data?

Simply put, categorical data are data that are naturally observed or more intuitively structured in categories, such as binary, multiple nominal, or ordinal data. In clinical research, categorical data are frequently binary (e.g., treatment success or failure, presence or absence of disease recurrence, reoperation). Examples of nominal data include categories which are not ordered, such as sex, eye color, or race and ethnicity. Ordinal data are not continuous, but able to be ordered, such as clothing size (e.g., small, medium, and large). Although analysis of continuous data will be reviewed in Chap. 3, ordinal data can include discrete variables with low maximum frequency counts or a finite number of responses, such as number of siblings or school grades (e.g., A, B, C, D, F).

© The Author(s), under exclusive license to Springer Nature Switzerland AG 2024

P. D. Fabricant, *Practical Clinical Research Design and Application*, https://doi.org/10.1007/978-3-031-58380-3_2

How Is Categorical Data Best Graphically Represented?

Bar charts are most commonly used to present categorical data counts or percentages, either as individual or stacked bars (Fig. 2.1). Pie charts should be discouraged, as it is difficult to visually compare angles or segments of a circle. Furthermore,

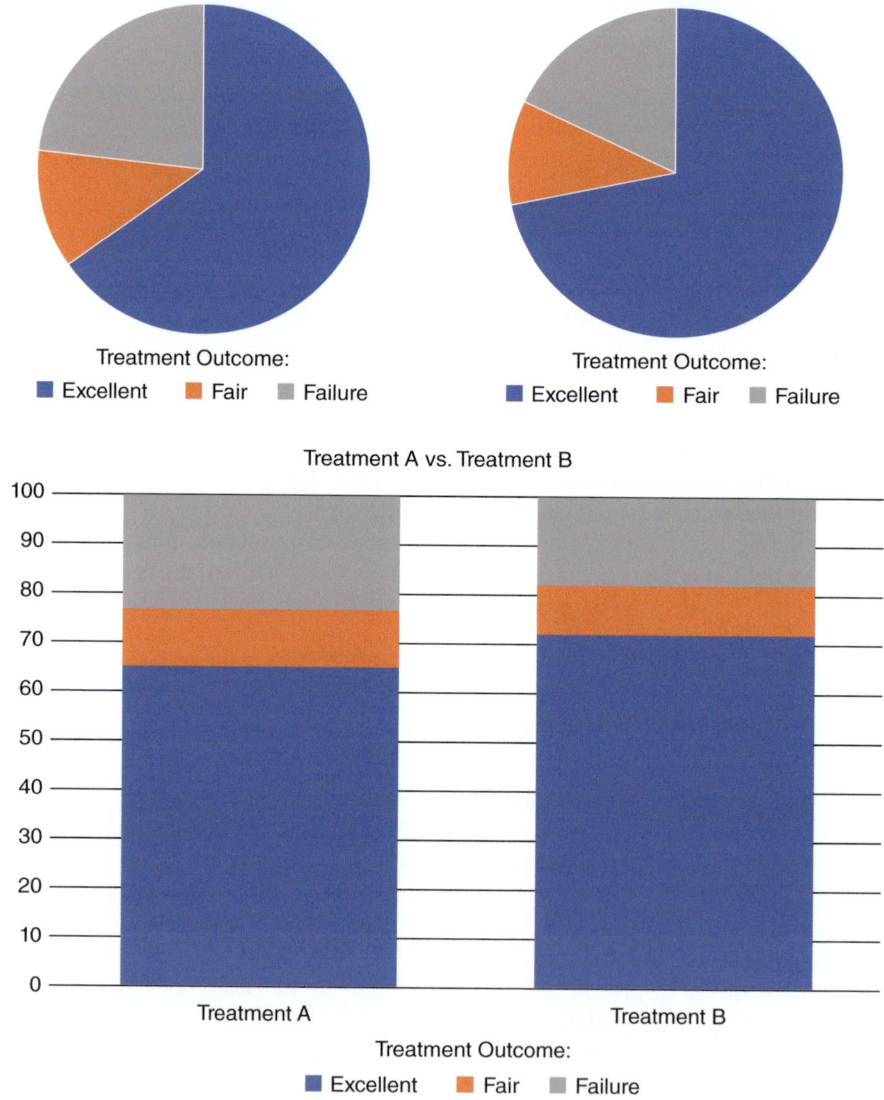

Fig. 2.1 A stacked bar chart is a better visual representation of proportions and categorical variables than a pie chart. The above charts show the same values for "Treatment A" and "Treatment B." It is much easier to visually compare treatment outcomes using stacked bar charts (bottom) than pie charts (top)

labels can be hard to match up to the respective "slice," and small percentages and differences can be challenging to convey. It is much easier to compare length or height, especially for small differences.

Bivariable Statistics for Categorical Data

Categorical data are most frequently arranged in 2×2 contingency tables, although they can be larger (e.g., $2 \times k$). Such data are analyzed using chi-squared or Fisher's exact tests. Chi-squared test is an approximation which assumes that the sample is large. When greater than 20% of the expected cell count is less than five, Fisher's exact test is used. While many statistical software packages will automatically calculate expected cell counts and indicate whether a chi-squared or Fisher's exact test is appropriate, calculating expected cell counts is straightforward and can be performed manually in order to choose the appropriate test.

Calculating Expected Cell Counts

In order to calculate expected cell counts, multiply the row and column totals associated with each cell, then divide by the grand total. An example is included below in Fig. 2.2.

	Disease (+)	Disease (−)	Total
Exposure (+)	A	B	A+B
Exposure (−)	C	D	C+D
Total	A+C	B+D	A+B+C+D

$$\text{Expected Cell Count A} = \frac{(A+B)\,(A+C)}{A+B+C+D}$$

$$\text{Expected Cell Count B} = \frac{(A+B)\,(B+D)}{A+B+C+D}$$

$$\text{Expected Cell Count C} = \frac{(C+D)\,(A+C)}{A+B+C+D}$$

$$\text{Expected Cell Count D} = \frac{(C+D)\,(B+D)}{A+B+C+D}$$

Fig. 2.2 Calculating expected cell counts are done using the margins and grand total. A, B, C, and D represent observed data. The margins (row and column totals) are calculated by adding up each row and column. Then, the corresponding margins are used to calculate expected cell counts as demonstrated above. For example, for cell A, it would be the row total (A + B) multiplied by the column total (A + C) divided by the grand total (A + B + C + D). This is done for each cell. If greater than 20% of the cells have an expected cell count of less than five, a Fisher's exact test is required. Otherwise, a chi-squared test is appropriate. In the case of a 2×2 table, all cells must have expected counts of ≥ 5 to perform a chi-squared test

	Treatment A	Treatment B	Treatment C	Total
Success	A	B	C	A+B+C
Failure	D	E	F	D+E+F
Total	A+D	B+E	C+F	A+B+C+D+E+F

Fig. 2.3 Post hoc pairwise analyses. In this example, a 3 × 2 table is shown evaluating three different treatments (A, B, and C) and whether they resulted in treatment success or failure. If all expected cell counts were ≥5 and the chi-squared test revealed a significant result ($P \leq 0.05$), it would be appropriate to do pairwise analyses. Frequently, this is done automatically within statistical software. It involves comparing the proportion of treatment success in Treatment A to Treatment B, Treatment B to Treatment C, and Treatment A to Treatment C to determine which treatment(s) demonstrate significantly higher (or lower) proportions of treatment success compared to others. It is important to note that in analyses requiring multiple comparisons, a Bonferroni correction is usually applied, adjusting the threshold of alpha (α) to a more stringent value equal to the original α divided by the number of comparisons being made. This example has a Bonferroni-corrected $\alpha = 0.05/3 = 0.017$

Post Hoc Pairwise Analyses

After the initial analysis (either chi-squared or Fisher's exact test), any $2 \times k$ table with $k > 2$ with a significant result ($P \leq 0.05$) should prompt post hoc pairwise analysis. This is because the initial result indicates that one proportion is different from at least one other proportion, but not which ones nor how many. After pairwise analyses are performed, the investigator can identify which groups are different from which other groups. It is important to understand why pairwise analyses are not done from the beginning and why an overall (also known as an "omnibus") test is performed. As discussed in detail in Chap. 4, alpha (α) is typically set to 0.05 to allow for 5% type I (false positive) error. Viewed another way, by random chance, 1 out of every 20 analyses may be significant. Therefore, one should aim to minimize multiple comparisons (i.e., "data dredging") whenever possible. In this case, that involves doing an omnibus test with multiple comparisons, only if the omnibus test demonstrates statistical significance. For a simple three group analysis, as illustrated in Fig. 2.3, the omnibus test is a single test, while pairwise comparisons would require three separate tests. The number of required analyses for pairwise testing only becomes greater with more groups.

Multivariable Statistics for Categorical Data: Logistic Regression

Multivariable statistics involve assessment of two or more independent explanatory variables to predict a single outcome. This is also referred to as "multiple regression." This should not be confused with "*multivariate* regression," which involves the use of two or more independent variables to predict multiple simultaneous outcomes [1].

The most commonly used multivariable statistical analysis with categorical data is logistic regression. Logistic regression (or "multiple logistic regression") is used to analyze the relationship(s) between two or more independent variables (may be categorical or continuous) and a single binary outcome. Explanatory variables are selected based on clinical judgment and those identified as significant in bivariable analyses for further testing in multiple logistic regression. When evaluated simultaneously in a model, each explanatory variable is examined while controlling for the other variables. This way, if an explanatory variable remains statistically significant in a multiple logistic regression model, it can be deemed an "independent predictor" of the outcome. If explanatory variables are found to be significant in bivariable analyses but not in multiple logistic regression, then their effect is thought to be due to the covariance of another variable. Finally, as discussed in Chap. 7, a variable is a confounder or mediator of a main effect if it is significantly associated with both the outcome and main explanatory variable being tested, and if controlling for that variable changes the magnitude of the main effect by 10% or more (Fig. 7.1).

Multiple logistic regression is represented by the formula:

$$\log\left(\frac{Y}{1-Y}\right) = \alpha + \beta_1 x_1 + \beta_2 x_2 + \beta_3 x_3 + \dots$$

where

$\log\left(\frac{Y}{1-Y}\right)$ is the log of the odds of the outcome event, Y, occurring.

α is the adjustment or random error term.

x_n is the explanatory variable linked to beta (β) in any given $\beta_n x_n$ term.

β_n is the amount by which a change in the associated x_n changes the log of the odds of the event occurring. This depends on the unit of measure of x, so that one unit change in x changes the log of the odds of the outcome by β. In the case of a continuous variable (e.g., age in years), it would represent one unit (e.g., year) of increasing age. In the case of a binary categorical variable (e.g., female sex), it would be the effect of female sex on the log of the odds of the outcome. In the case of an ordinal categorical variable (e.g., school grade level), it would represent the effect of each additional unit (e.g., year in school) on the log of the odds of outcome. A positive β value indicates a direct relationship (increasing the odds of outcome with increasing units of x), while a negative β value indicates an inverse relationship (decreasing the odds of outcome with increasing units of x).

One important caveat to consider when constructing a multiple logistic regression model is to ensure that there are not too many explanatory variables being evaluated in a single analysis. This is because if a model has too many predictors, it will model random error in the data rather than solely the relationship among the variables of interest. This leads to "overfitting" or falsely high values of model fit (R-squared), and, consequently, a lower predictive ability of the model. Therefore, it is commonly accepted practice that there should be no more than one explanatory variable per 20 "events" being studied [2]. For example, if the binary outcome under investigation is the presence or absence of postoperative infection and an investigator wants to test seven independent variables, there should be at least $7 \times 20 = 140$ infection cases in the dataset, regardless of how many patients are in the overall study cohort.

Conclusion

In summary, many predictor variables and outcome measurements in clinical research are categorical. Categorical outcomes are best displayed as bar or stacked bar charts. They should be analyzed using two-proportion z-tests, Fisher's exact tests, and/or chi-squared tests with post hoc pairwise comparisons as needed for multiple groups when the initial screening test is significant. For multiple predictor variables and a dichotomous outcome, logistic regression is the appropriate regression analysis.

As a primer, this text reviewed the fundamental concepts of categorical data analysis. However, there are several important topics that are beyond the scope of this book. These include the use of continuity correction, assessing for interaction, matched pair analysis, n x m contingency tables, ordinal logistic and Poisson regression, among others. Further in-depth reading on these and other categorical data analysis topics should include important work by Alan Agresti and Tamás Rudas [3, 4].

References

1. Kolin DA, Landy DC, Watkins A, et al. The terms "multivariate" and "multivariable" are used incorrectly and interchangeably in Orthopaedic publications: should we care about the distinction? J Bone Joint Surg Am. 2022;105:896–9. https://doi.org/10.2106/JBJS.22.00598.
2. Austin PC, Steyerberg EW. Events per variable (EPV) and the relative performance of different strategies for estimating the out-of-sample validity of logistic regression models. Stat Methods Med Res. 2017;26:796–808. https://doi.org/10.1177/0962280214558972.
3. Agresti A. Categorical data analysis. Hoboken, NJ: John Wiley & Sons; 2012.
4. Rudas T. Lectures on categorical data analysis. New York, NY: Springer; 2018.

Chapter 3
Comparative Statistics: Continuous Data

Introduction

Continuous data is ubiquitous in clinical research. Physiologic variables (e.g., height, weight, temperature, body mass index, age) are frequently used as continuous variables. Many outcome variables are continuous as well. Clinical outcome scales, such as Patient-Reported Outcomes Measurement Information System (PROMIS), volume of blood loss, and pain medication requirement (reported as morphine milligram equivalent), are a few examples.

This chapter will review the concepts around reporting and analyzing continuous data including bivariable analyses (such as t-tests, ANOVA, Pearson's correlation, and their nonparametric counterparts) and multivariable analyses (e.g., multiple linear regression). Although the formulas for calculating test statistics are beyond the scope of this book, this chapter will provide insight into the concepts of continuous data analysis, explaining how to select the appropriate test and interpret research reporting continuous data analyses.

What Is Continuous Data?

Continuous data are data that can take on any value within a finite or infinite interval. With continuous data, values can be added, subtracted, and do not have any fixed values. Examples include age, height, body mass index, temperature, and many clinical outcome scores (such as those with scores ranging from 0 to 100). Some ordinal data with equal intervals between each level can be presented as continuous, for example, school grade (ordinal) versus years of schooling (continuous).

P. D. Fabricant, *Practical Clinical Research Design and Application*, https://doi.org/10.1007/978-3-031-58380-3_3

Continuous variables are occasionally categorized in clinical research. Categorization can facilitate comparison of new data with prior studies (e.g., a prior study categorized a patient body temperature variable as febrile or afebrile, rather than in degrees Celsius). In predictive modeling, categorization of predictor variables can make it easier for clinicians to interpret and apply study findings to inform clinical decisions. Additionally, there may be physiologic reasons for categorizing continuous variables. For example, a one-unit increase in oxygen saturation from 40% to 41% is unlikely to be the same as a similar increase from 98% to 99%, as the former values are not compatible with life. In this case, categorization of oxygen saturation, which technically can range from 0 to 100, into a categorical variable may not only be intuitive, but clinically sound. It is important to emphasize that categorization of continuous variables should not be done arbitrarily. Full analysis of data in continuous variable format should be performed first and should justify the result that is illustrated by a simpler categorical representation [1]. Categorization must also follow clinically meaningful cutoffs (e.g., pediatric or adult age categories in orthopedics based on skeletal age), established laboratory reference values, or receiver operating characteristic (ROC) analysis (see Chap. 5). In some models, categorization can be performed by creating even groups based on the continuous data (e.g., divide categories above and below the median, or into quartiles, quintiles, etc.); however, this is less intuitive and therefore has less clinical utility than categorization by clinical meaningful cutoffs. Finally, categorization of continuous variables increases degrees of freedom in a model, and therefore, usually results in loss of statistical power unless sample size is increased [2].

How Is Continuous Data Best Graphically Represented?

Boxplots (Fig. 3.1), scatterplots (Fig. 3.2), and histograms (Fig. 3.3) are most frequently used to graphically represent continuous data. Bar graphs may also be used to graphically represent summarized continuous data between groups (Fig. 3.4).

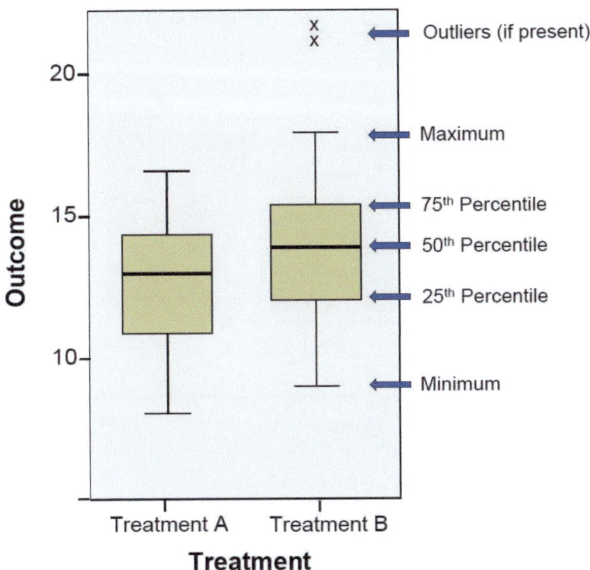

Fig. 3.1 A boxplot is a graphical depiction of numerical data through their quartiles. The typical plot includes both a "box" and "whiskers." As noted in figure, the box is defined by the 75th percentile at its upper limit, the 25th percentile at its lower limit, and an additional horizontal line denotes the median (or 50th percentile). The whiskers extending above and below represent the maximum and minimum data values, respectively, and must end at an observed data point. Whiskers may be portrayed in one of two ways: either as the true maximum and minimum (including any outliers) or using the 1.5 interquartile range (IQR) rule. In the 1.5 IQR rule, whiskers are drawn from the upper and lower quartile a distance of 1.5 times the IQR to the farthest observed data point in that range. Additional outlier data are drawn in individually. In this example, a continuous outcome score (vertical axis) is being compared between two treatments being studied (horizontal axis)

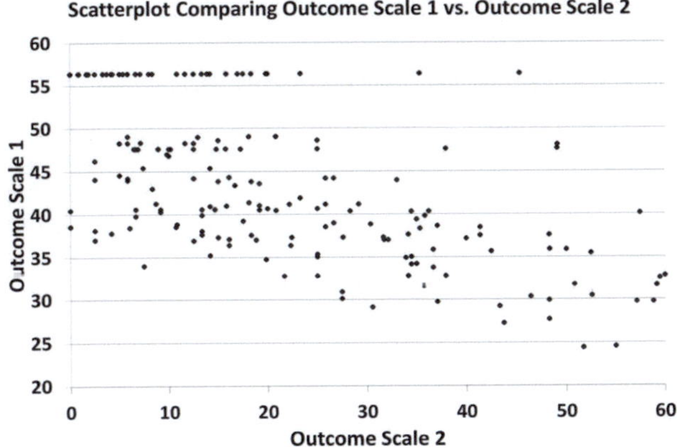

Fig. 3.2 Scatterplots graphically depict the relationship between two continuous variables by marking a point on the plot area corresponding to an individual participant's data for each variable. In this example, if each participant completed two outcome scales, each participant's score is plotted at the intersection of their scores on each outcome scale. Correlation analyses can be performed, and lines of best fit may be added to the plot

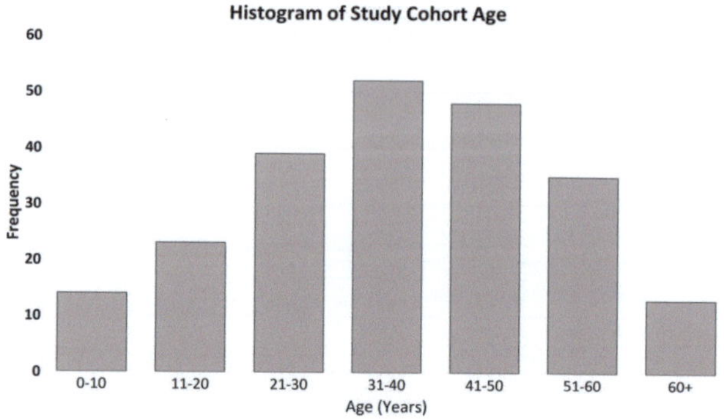

Fig. 3.3 Histograms can be used to graphically depict the frequency distribution of a continuous variable, which has been classified into "bins" or ranges. This example depicts the frequency distribution of participant ages in a study cohort (continuous variable but presented in 10-year bins)

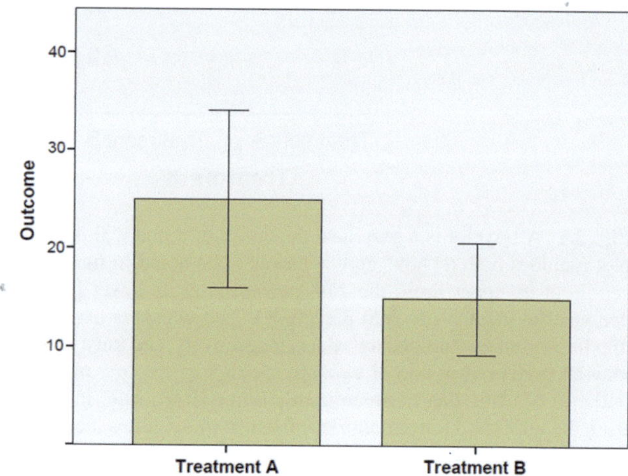

Fig. 3.4 Bar graphs summarize groupwise continuous data. In this example, the bar heights represent the group means of a continuous outcome between two treatments being studied, and the error bars extend one standard deviation above and below the means

Bivariable Statistics for Continuous Data

When deciding the appropriate test for continuous data, one must understand three elements about the data structure: how many categories are being studied, whether the data being compared is between-patients (e.g., two different cohorts) or within-patients (e.g., repeated measures in the same patient), and whether the data are normally or not normally distributed (Chap. 1). Then, the appropriate test may be selected from Table 3.1.

Post Hoc Pairwise Analyses

For data with greater than two comparison groups, after the initial analysis (e.g., ANOVA) is performed, a significant result ($P \leq 0.05$) should prompt a post hoc pairwise analysis. The initial result only indicates that one group's median or mean is different from at least one other group, but does not identify which one(s). If a

Table 3.1 Selecting the correct statistical test for analyzing continuous data

Number of categories/cohorts	Between vs. within patients	Parametric test	Non-parametric test
2	Between patients	Independent samples t-test	Mann-Whitney U test
2	Within patients	Paired samples t-test	Wilcoxon signed-rank test
>2	Between patients	One-way ANOVA	Kruskal-Wallis test
>2	Within patients	Repeated measures ANOVA	Friedman test
Correlation between 2 continuous variables	Each pair of variables is plotted within patients, then correlation analyzed between patients	Pearson's r	Spearman's rho (ρ)

difference is found, pairwise analyses are performed to identify which groups are different from which other groups. It is important to understand why pairwise analyses are not done from the beginning (e.g., multiple t-tests among subgroups rather than a single exploratory ANOVA). As discussed in detail in Chap. 4, alpha (α) is typically set to 0.05 to allow for 5% type I (false positive) error. Viewed another way, by random chance, one out of every 20 analyses may be significant. Therefore, one should aim to minimize multiple comparisons (i.e., "data dredging") whenever possible. In this case, that involves doing an omnibus test with multiple comparisons only in the event that the omnibus test demonstrates statistical significance. For a simple three group analysis, the omnibus test is a single test, while pairwise comparisons require three separate tests. The number of required analyses for pairwise testing only becomes greater with more groups.

Similar to categorical analyses, a Bonferroni correction for multiple comparisons is usually applied by adjusting the threshold of α to a more stringent value equal to the original α divided by the number of comparisons being made. In the case of three pairwise comparisons, a Bonferroni-corrected alpha would be $\alpha = 0.05/3 = 0.017$.

Multivariable Statistics for Continuous Data: Linear Regression

Multivariable regression involves inclusion of several independent explanatory variables to predict a single outcome. This should not be confused with "multivariate regression" which involves the use of several independent variables to predict two or more simultaneous outcomes [3].

The customary multivariable statistical analysis for continuous outcomes is linear regression. Linear regression (also known as "multiple linear regression" or, simply, "multiple regression") is used to analyze the relationship(s) between two or more independent variables (may be categorical or continuous) and a single continuous outcome. Explanatory variables are selected using clinical judgment and the statistics outlined above to find bivariable associations that can be tested further in multiple linear regression. When evaluated simultaneously, each explanatory variable is examined while controlling for all other variables in the model. If an explanatory variable remains statistically significant in a regression model, it can be deemed an "independent predictor" of the outcome. If explanatory variables are found to be significant in bivariable analyses but not in multiple regression, then their effect is thought to be due to the covariance of another variable. Finally, as discussed in Chap. 7, a variable is considered a confounder or mediator if it meets both of the following criteria. First, it is significantly associated with both the outcome and main explanatory variable, and second, controlling for that variable in regression analysis changes the magnitude of the main effect (i.e., β) by 10% or greater (see Fig. 7.1).

Multiple linear regression is represented by the formula:

$$Y = \alpha + \beta_1 x_1 + \beta_2 x_2 + \beta_3 x_3 + \ldots$$

where

Y is the predicted value of the outcome, which is a continuous variable.

α is the random error term or adjustment, which is also the Y-intercept.

x_n is the explanatory variable linked to beta in any given $\beta_n x_n$ term.

β_n is the amount by which a change in the associated x_n changes the continuous outcome variable.

Of note, this interpretation depends on the unit of measure of x, so that one-unit change in x changes the outcome (Y) by β. In the case of a continuous independent variable (e.g., age in years), it would represent one unit (e.g., year) of increasing age on the outcome. In the case of a binary categorical independent variable (e.g., female sex), it would be the effect of female sex on the outcome. In the case of an ordinal categorical predictor variable (e.g., school grade), it would represent the effect of each additional unit (e.g., year in school) on the outcome. A positive β value indicates a direct relationship (increasing Y with increasing units of x), while a negative β value indicates an inverse relationship (decreasing Y with increasing units of x).

Oftentimes, an R^2 value (the coefficient of determination) is reported alongside a regression analysis. This is a value from 0 to 1 and indicates how well the regression model fits the data, specifically the proportion of the variability in outcome that is explained by the dependent variables in the model. For example, if an R^2 value is 0.81, then 81% of the variation in Y is accounted for by the independent variables (x_n) included in the model.

Conclusion

In summary, understanding continuous data analysis is imperative when conducting and reading clinical research. Continuous outcomes are optimally displayed as boxplots, scatterplots, histograms, or bar graphs. They are best analyzed using t-tests, ANOVA, or their nonparametric counterparts. Post hoc pairwise comparisons are used as needed for multiple groups when the initial screening test is significant. When there are multiple predictor variables, linear regression is used to identify independent predictors of a continuous outcome.

References

1. Gelman A, Park DK. Splitting a predictor at the upper quarter or third and the lower quarter or third. Am Stat. 2009;63:1–8. https://doi.org/10.1198/tast.2009.0001.
2. Irwin JR, McClelland GH. Negative consequences of dichotomizing continuous predictor variables. J Mark Res. 2003;40:366–71. https://doi.org/10.1509/jmkr.40.3.366.19237.
3. Kolin DA, Landy DC, Watkins A, et al. The terms "multivariate" and "multivariable" are used incorrectly and interchangeably in orthopaedic publications: should we care about the distinction? J Bone Joint Surg Am. 2022;105:896–9. https://doi.org/10.2106/JBJS.22.00598.

Chapter 4
Statistical Power and Power Calculations

Introduction

The interplay among statistical power, the performance of power calculations, and the number of patients needed for a study is crucial in the design and planning of clinical research studies. Statistical power refers to the probability of finding a statistically significant result when a true effect exists in the population under investigation. In other words, it measures the ability of a study to detect the existence of a true effect. Power calculations are done a priori (prior to beginning a study). This allows investigators to determine the appropriate sample size required for detection of a specified effect size with a given level of confidence.

Power is influenced by several factors, including the effect size (magnitude of the effect being studied), the desired power level (usually set at 0.8 or higher), the significance level (typically set at 0.05), the sample size, and the variability of the data. The larger the sample size, the greater the statistical power of the study. A larger sample size reduces the random variability in the data and increases the chances of detecting a true effect. Conversely, a smaller sample size may result in lower statistical power and a higher likelihood of failing to detect a real effect, even if one exists.

Just as it is essential to understand the minimum number of study participants required to adequately power a study, it is important to avoid maximizing the sample size indefinitely to increase statistical power. This is neither appropriate nor practical. In addition to the practical limitations of an enormous study sample, ethical considerations and financial constraints must be considered when determining the appropriate sample size for a study.

P. D. Fabricant, *Practical Clinical Research Design and Application*, https://doi.org/10.1007/978-3-031-58380-3_4

Selecting a Primary Outcome of Interest

Although studies may be designed to investigate a multitude of outcomes, research questions should be formulated with a primary outcome of interest upon which the study is also powered. A primary outcome variable should be precisely measurable, valid, and clinically meaningful to clinicians and researchers. Particularly with patient-reported outcome measures (PROMs), it is important to choose outcomes that are valid for the clinical condition being investigated in the study population of interest. This ensures that those outcome measures are appropriate and applicable to those research participants. Alternatively, hard outcomes (typically binary, e.g., death, infection, reinjury, treatment success or failure) are usually not specifically validated in a cohort or condition of interest but are clinically meaningful nonetheless. They may also be used as a primary outcome variable upon which a power calculation may be performed.

Statistical Power and Power Calculations

When preparing to perform a prospective study, particularly a randomized controlled trial (RCT), the investigator must perform a power analysis in order to determine the number of study participants required for enrollment. Once there is a decision on a primary outcome of interest upon which to power the study, the investigator must set error thresholds and identify study characteristics to perform a power calculation and determine the number of research participants required to adequately power the proposed study. While sample size is determined by a power calculation performed on the primary outcome, power analyses for secondary outcomes may also be performed to ensure that there will be adequate power to analyze them.

Error thresholds include alpha (α) and beta (β):

- **Alpha (α)**: Threshold is typically set to 0.05 to allow for 5% type I error (Fig. 4.1). This may be adjusted to stricter values such as 0.01 or 0.005 when investigating new discoveries, drugs, or interventions where a positive result might change clinical practice. This further limits type I error and reduces the rate of false positives which are of growing concern in clinical research [1]. Decreasing alpha will increase the number of participants needed for enrollment.
- **Beta (β)**: Threshold is typically set to 0.2 to allow for 20% type II error and 80% power (Fig. 4.1). This may be decreased to 0.1 (thereby increasing to 90% power) to decrease the risk of type II error (false negatives). Decreasing beta (and increasing power) will increase the number of participants needed for enrollment.

If the null hypothesis is rejected and there is a true difference between groups (Fig. 4.1, top left box), then this is a true positive result with the probability $(1-\alpha)$. When α is set to 0.05, that results in a 95% probability that rejecting the null hypothesis is the correct study outcome and a 5% probability that the null hypothesis gets

	TRUE Difference Between Groups	FALSE No Difference Between Groups
Null Hypothesis Rejected	Correct Study Outcome True Positive Probability = 1-α	Type I Error False Positive Probability = α
Null Hypothesis NOT Rejected	Type II Error False Negative Probability = β	Correct Study Outcome True Negative Probability = 1-β

Fig. 4.1 The interplay between true differences between groups or no difference between groups and rejection or no rejection of the null hypothesis

rejected where there is no difference between groups (false positive, type I error, top right box).

If the null hypothesis is *not* rejected and there is no difference between groups (Fig. 4.1, bottom right box), then this is a true negative result with the probability (1-β). When β is set to 0.2, that results in an 80% probability that not rejecting the null hypothesis is the correct study outcome and a 20% probability that the null hypothesis is not rejected when there is in fact a difference between groups (false negative, type II error, bottom left box).

Additional data required for the power analysis and their effect on number of required study participants are:

- **Effect size of the primary outcome of interest**: Effect size is the magnitude of difference in the primary outcome between groups. This is frequently set as the minimal clinically important difference in the outcome. Powering a study to detect a smaller effect size requires a greater number of study participants than testing for a larger difference between groups (Fig. 4.2).
- **Expected distribution of the primary outcome of interest**: The expected variance or standard deviation of an outcome can affect the number of study participants required for enrollment. A greater distribution of the primary outcome of interest (e.g., wider standard deviation or variance) would require enrollment of more participants to discern a treatment effect of the intervention compared with controls (Fig. 4.2).
- **Number of treatment arms**: More treatment arms/groups require a greater number of study participants to attain the same amount of statistical power.
- **Proportion of study participants that will be assigned to each treatment arm**: When study participants are more evenly distributed among groups (i.e., closer to 1:1 ratio), fewer are needed for enrollment. Conversely, when the group ratios are more imbalanced (e.g., 2:1, 3:1, etc.), a greater number of total participants are required for enrollment. For instance, a study with 2:1 ratio of study participants in an RCT with two treatment arms will require a greater number of total participants than a study with 1:1 ratio of participants.

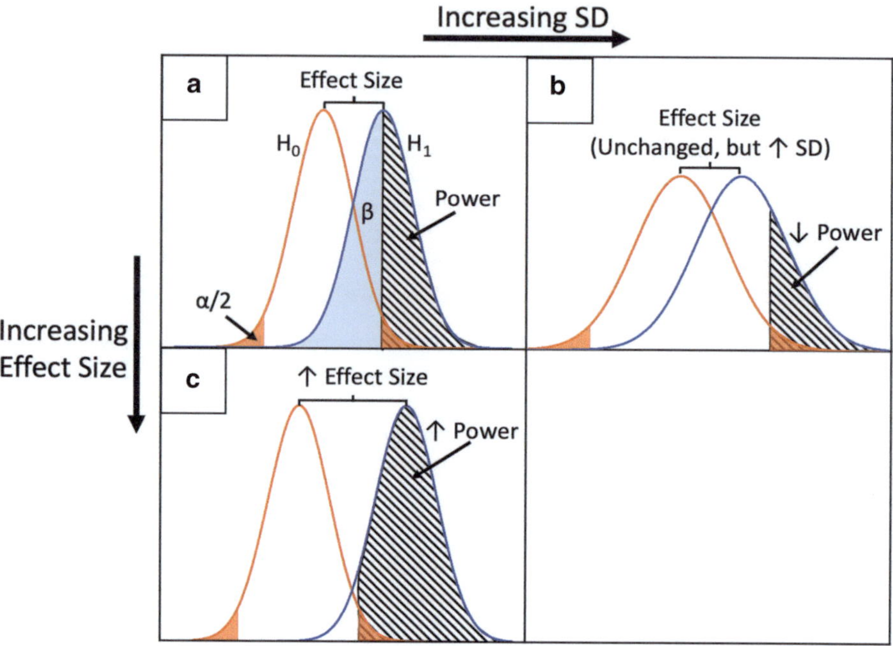

Fig. 4.2 This figure demonstrates the impact of changing the expected effect size and/or standard deviation (SD) on power and, as a result, the number of study participants needed to enroll. In this figure, H_0 represents the distribution of the null hypothesis and H_1 is the distribution of the alternate hypothesis. Power (hatched area) is the area under the H_1 curve to the right of a cutoff line at the upper $\alpha/2$ area under the H_0 curve. Because expected effect size and SD alter curve shape and the relationships between the two curves, they can both affect power. As the expected effect size increases (**panel a** to **panel c**), the distribution of H_0 and H_1 moves farther apart. Due to the decreased data overlap, there is increased power (hatched area under the H_1 curve to the right of the upper $\alpha/2$ area under the H_0 curve increases). As a result, with greater power, fewer study participants are needed for enrollment. Conversely, as data distribution or SD increases (**panel a** to **panel b**), there is increased overlap of the curves. In this scenario, power decreases, and the required number of enrolled participants increases as a result

- **Expected loss to follow-up**: Once a power calculation is performed to determine the appropriate number of study participants for analysis, investigators must consider adjusting for: eligible patients who are missed, eligible patients who decline enrollment, and patients who enroll but are lost to follow-up. Based on their own or others' similar work with the population, intervention, or outcome(s) of interest, investigators should enroll a greater number of study participants than that calculated from their power analysis. This ensures there is an appropriate number for enrollment to account for participants that drop out or are lost to follow-up. This additional "buffer" is typically smaller for studies requiring shorter follow-up and larger when the potential for drop out is high (e.g., longer follow-up interval or a transient patient population who may be more easily lost to follow-up).

Post Hoc Power Calculations

Post hoc power calculations deserve special mention. They have become increasingly popular to report in retrospective investigations or cross-sectional studies that use all available patient data and, upon completion of data analysis, find a negative result. To justify the negative finding, some investigators use the study data to report power after the study has been completed. Typically, this is done by calculating the "observed power" based on the calculated test statistic for the primary analysis. However, this is never appropriate because the observed test statistic and, by derivation, the significance level (p-value) would also determine the observed power [2]. Furthermore, post hoc power analysis relies on effect sizes based on observed data. These effect sizes may not accurately represent the true effect in the population, as they are influenced by sample-specific characteristics and random variability. Correctly performed power calculations rely on the effect size specification of the underlying population, not just the study sample. By using the observed data to perform a post hoc power analysis, an investigator predicates the analysis on the likely incorrect assumption that the effect size in the study sample is identical to the effect size in the population from which it was drawn [3]. Thus, the calculated power may not be considered a reliable indicator of the true power of the study [2].

Given these faults and limitations, it is inappropriate to rely on post hoc power analysis as a reliable indicator of study quality or statistical power. Instead, as described earlier in this chapter, power calculations should only be performed during the planning stage of a study. They should be based on reasonable population effect size estimates from available data and desired power levels to determine the appropriate sample size, never as an afterthought. This ensures that an adequate sample size is used from the outset. If all available patient data is being used for a retrospective study (e.g., due to a rare condition or intervention), then no power calculation is performed. But if a negative result (e.g., no difference) is observed, then the possibility of a false negative (type II error) must be considered. With rare conditions or interventions, it may be more appropriate to report these as a case series or case report (Chap. 12).

Conclusion

In summary, statistical power, the precise execution of an a priori power calculation, and the appropriate number of patients needed for a study are tightly interconnected. Power calculations estimate the required sample size to achieve the desired level of statistical power. This affects the ability of a study to detect a true effect. Proper consideration of these factors is essential in designing studies that can produce reliable and meaningful results.

References

1. Benjamin DJ, Berger JO, Johannesson M, et al. Redefine statistical significance. Nat Hum Behav. 2018;2:6–10. https://doi.org/10.1038/s41562-017-0189-z.
2. Hoenig JM, Heisey DM. The abuse of power: the pervasive fallacy of power calculations for data analysis. Am Stat. 2001;55:1–6. https://doi.org/10.1198/000313001300339897.
3. Zumbo BD, Hubley AM. A note on misconceptions concerning prospective and retrospective power. Statistician. 1998;47:385–8. https://doi.org/10.1111/1467-9884.00139.

Chapter 5
Characteristics of a Diagnostic Test: Sensitivity, Specificity, Positive Predictive Value, and Negative Predictive Value

Introduction

Diagnostic tests are ubiquitous in research, as well as in clinical medicine and surgery. Most commonly, diagnostic tests produce a result with a continuous value (e.g., serum concentration of a detectable marker) from which threshold values are established to interpret the test as being either "positive" or "negative." When utilizing diagnostic tests, it is important to understand the contributing factors that differentiate the result as being positive or negative: sensitivity, specificity, positive predictive value (PPV), and negative predictive value (NPV). Each of these concepts are illustrated below.

Each calculation is performed using the contents of a 2 × 2 table (Fig. 5.1).

	Disease (+)	Disease (-)
Test (+)	A (True Positive)	B (False Positive)
Test (-)	C (False Negative)	D (True Negative)

Fig. 5.1 Standard 2 × 2 table from which sensitivity, specificity, PPV, and NPV can be calculated
- (A) represents study patients who are "true positives," those who have a positive diagnostic test and have the disease or condition.
- (B) represents study patients who are "false positives," those who have a positive diagnostic test but do not have the disease or condition.
- (C) represents study patients who are "false negatives," those who have a negative diagnostic test but have the disease or condition.
- (D) represents study patients who are "true negatives," those who have a negative diagnostic test and do not have the disease or condition

P. D. Fabricant, *Practical Clinical Research Design and Application*, https://doi.org/10.1007/978-3-031-58380-3_5

Sensitivity

Sensitivity, a measure of a test's ability to correctly identify as many disease positive patients as possible, is the proportion of patients who have the disease and test positive. In other words, a test with perfect sensitivity will identify all of the patients who have the disease and will not have any false negatives. This is important in a screening test designed to capture all patients who have the disease, even if some who do not have the disease are falsely identified as positive. To that end, tests with high sensitivity are good at *ruling out* disease, so that those who test negative do not need further testing ("SnOUT"). One example of a highly sensitive test for colon cancer is fecal occult blood testing. This non-invasive, inexpensive, and rapid test detects microscopic blood present in stool, which may be a sign of colon cancer. If fecal occult blood testing is negative, it is unlikely that colon cancer is present. However, some patients may have a positive fecal occult blood test but not have colon cancer (false positive).

In the above 2 × 2 table, sensitivity is calculated as:

$$\text{Sensitivity} = \frac{\text{True positives}}{\text{All patients with disease}} = \frac{A}{A+C}$$

Specificity

Specificity, a measure of a test's ability to correctly identify as many disease-negative patients as possible, is the proportion of patients without the disease who test negative. In other words, a test with perfect specificity will identify all the patients who do not have the disease and will not have any false positives. To that end, tests with high specificity are good at *ruling in* disease ("SpIN"). This is important in a confirmatory test that might lead to more invasive testing and/or treatment. To continue with the above example, colonoscopy is a highly specific test that may be used to confirm a diagnosis of colon cancer though direct visualization and tissue biopsy. However, this test is invasive and expensive. Therefore, it is generally only performed in patients with a positive fecal occult blood test or who have other risk factors for colon cancer.

In the above 2 × 2 table, specificity is calculated as:

$$\text{Specificity} = \frac{\text{True negatives}}{\text{All patients without disease}} = \frac{D}{B+D}$$

Positive Predictive Value

Positive predictive value (PPV) represents the chances that a positive test result is a true positive. It is calculated as the proportion of all test-positive patients who have the disease. In other words, for a test with a perfect PPV, a positive result will be a true positive and there will be no false positives. Unlike sensitivity and specificity, which are inherent characteristics of the diagnostic test that are unaffected by prevalence of disease in the population, PPV increases as the prevalence of disease (e.g., pretest probability) increases. An illustrative example of a test with 50% sensitivity and 50% specificity is a coin flip. The chances that a coin flip resulting in heads represents a true disease positive is based solely on the pretest probability of disease. If the disease prevalence is 95% in the population of interest, the chances of heads being met with a true positive is much higher than if the pretest probability was 10% in the population of interest. The higher the pretest probability, the greater the PPV, and the lower the NPV.

$$PPV = \frac{\text{True positives}}{\text{All patients who test positive}} = \frac{A}{A+B}$$

Negative Predictive Value

Negative predictive value (NPV) represents the chances that a negative test result is a true negative. It is calculated as the proportion of all test-negative patients that do not have the disease. In other words, for a test with perfect NPV, a negative result will be a true negative and there will be no false negatives. As is the case with PPV, NPV is affected by the prevalence of disease in the population of interest (e.g., pretest probability). As pretest probability decreases (indicated by a lower disease prevalence), NPV increases (conversely, PPV decreases).

$$NPV = \frac{\text{True negatives}}{\text{All patients who test negative}} = \frac{D}{C+D}$$

Accuracy Versus Precision

Test accuracy and precision are graphically depicted in Fig. 5.2. For a test to be clinically useful, it must first demonstrate acceptable precision. In other words, repeated testing must produce consistent results. Second, the test must be accurate, meaning that the results of the test must represent the "true values" of the clinical condition. A test that is precise but not accurate (Fig. 5.2, top right panel) may be recalibrated such that the values produced can be both precise and accurate. However, if a test lacks precision (also known as reliability or reproducibility), it has an unpredictable output. Therefore, it cannot be recalibrated and is unlikely to be clinically useful.

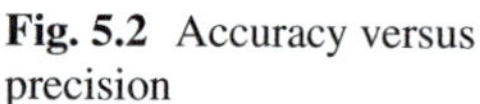

Fig. 5.2 Accuracy versus precision

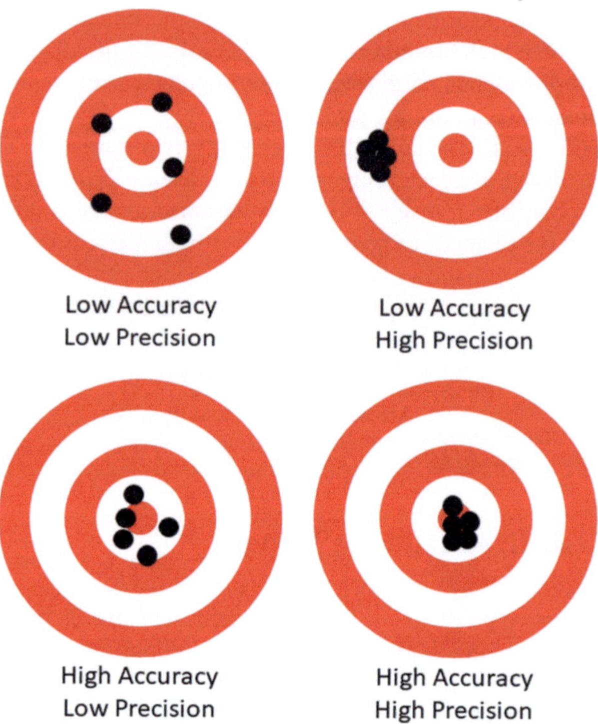

How Are Test Threshold Values Determined? ROC Curves

Threshold values for diagnostic tests are established through the use of receiver operating characteristic (ROC) curves. The ROC curve is a graphical method for displaying the performance of a diagnostic test. It is utilized below to illustrate the overall discriminative capacity of a test and to show how threshold cutoffs can be chosen.

To generate an ROC curve, a cohort of patients is formed by those who are known by some gold standard to be positive or negative for disease and who also have undergone the diagnostic test being evaluated (generating a continuous output). An ROC plot is generated by assessing each possible test output threshold and creating a plot based on the sensitivity and (1-specificity) as if each possible value was used as the threshold to determine the condition of interest (Fig. 5.3). The concordance statistic (or "C-statistic") is the area under the curve (AUC). It is a quantitative measure of test accuracy.

Figure 5.3 demonstrates a ROC curve. "Sensitivity" is displayed on the *y*-axis and "1-specificity" (the false positive rate) on the *x*-axis, both as a number between 0 and 1, represent a range of 0–100%. Therefore, if there was a perfect threshold value (e.g., 100% sensitivity and 100% specificity), the corresponding value would be plotted in the upper left corner of the plot. The area below the diagonal line (a) represents an AUC of 0.5, which would be a test that is no better than chance. A

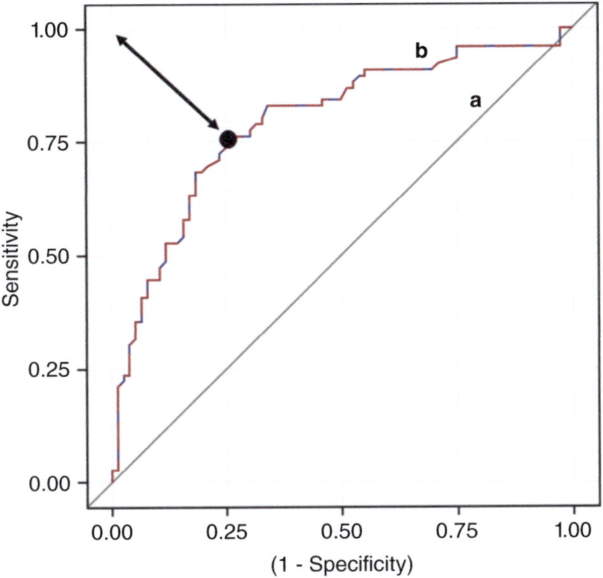

Fig. 5.3 Receiver operating characteristic (ROC) curve illustrating the characteristics of a diagnostic test

perfect test (with a threshold value in the upper left corner) would have an AUC of 1.0. The AUC is used to determine the discriminative capacity of a test. Generally, values of 0.7–0.8 are considered acceptable, 0.8–0.9 are considered excellent, and >0.9 are considered outstanding [1]. The curve (b) represents the sensitivity and (1-specificity) values of various possible thresholds for a positive or negative test result. The Youden Index is defined as the point in the ROC curve with the shortest distance to the upper left-hand corner (double ended arrow). It is used to determine the optimal cutoff value in the ROC curve (black dot) which maximizes sensitivity and specificity. In the above example, the test has a sensitivity of 75% and a specificity of (1–0.25) = 75%.

After confirming that the test has acceptable discriminative capacity (e.g., AUC $\geq$ 0.7), the Youden Index is calculated for each threshold value on the curve and equals sensitivity + specificity - 1 (maximum score is 1). Selecting the cutoff with the highest Youden Index appropriately minimizes overall diagnostic error, but assumes that false negative and false positive results have the same clinical consequence. Instead, what is considered acceptable for each test and cutoff values for a positive/negative result must match the risk tolerance of getting a false positive or false negative result. Consequently, an investigator may choose a cutoff value on either side of the Youden index that prioritizes specificity or sensitivity because a perfect text with 100% sensitivity and 100% specificity may not be possible. For instance, if the test is meant to be a screening test for a serious disease where it is of the utmost importance not to miss any potential positive cases, then one might consider maximizing sensitivity (in order to identify all potential cases) even at the risk of sacrificing specificity (e.g., may get some false positives). This may be then paired with a confirmatory test that has a high specificity for the disease. One well-known example of this is the process of testing for Human Immunodeficiency Virus (HIV). First, a blood sample is obtained, and an enzyme-linked immunosorbent assay (ELISA) test is performed which has a high sensitivity for HIV (albeit with less optimal specificity). If the ELISA is negative, no further testing is performed on the sample because of the high sensitivity. However, if the ELISA is positive, then a Western Blot or HIV differentiation assay is performed (each with a high specificity) to confirm the positive result. If both the ELISA and confirmatory tests are positive, then the patient is considered to have tested positive for HIV. If the ELISA is positive and the confirmatory test is negative, then the ELISA is considered to be a false positive. In this manner, a combination of multiple tests with varying sensitivity and specificity may be performed in a series to maximize diagnostic accuracy.

Reference

1. Hosmer DW, Lemeshow S, Sturdivant RX. Applied logistic regression. 2nd ed. Hoboken, NJ: John Wiley & Sons; 2013. p. 160–4.

Chapter 6
Statistical Bias

Introduction

Clinical research is performed with a representative cohort of research participants that are drawn from a larger population. The results from the sample cohort
are then generalized back to the entire population of interest. At each step of performing a clinical research study (patient identification, patient enrollment and
group assignment, data collection, data analysis and interpretation, and study publication), systematic error may lead to differences between the true condition of a
population and the estimates or judgments about that population. These biases are
common and can result in the skewing of results and incorrect assessment of a
population of interest.

It is important to emphasize that statistical bias results from any of several possible systematic errors of which the most common are described in this chapter.
Conversely, random error (also known as random variation or "noise") is inherent to
all data but does not cause statistical bias.

Finally, after noting any potential biases in a study, it is vital to understand precisely how they might affect the study data and results. Statistical bias may skew
results both toward the null hypothesis (i.e., causing a type II error—where no association is identified when one does exist) or away from the null hypothesis (i.e.,
causing a type I error—where an association is identified but one does not exist).
Recognition of the direction in which bias may skew results is essential when drawing conclusions from study data.

Included in this chapter are several common sources of bias in clinical research
presented with their effect on study results, as well as potential solutions to avoid
them or mitigate their impact.

P. D. Fabricant, *Practical Clinical Research Design and Application*,
https://doi.org/10.1007/978-3-031-58380-3_6

Selection Bias

Selection bias, one of the most common forms of statistical bias in clinical research, can happen during any phase of a study in which patients are being identified, assigned, or analyzed. In the earliest phases of study design, selection bias may occur when applying inclusion and exclusion criteria during study enrollment. Investigators must ensure that inclusion and exclusion criteria generate a study sample which is representative of the population of interest and does not systematically oversample or exclude some portion of the population.

In an experimental study, randomization of treatment group assignment minimizes the risk of selection bias. Given a large enough sample, there should be an equal distribution of patient characteristics (both those that are measurable and those that are not measurable) between each group. In an observational study, this becomes more challenging, as the investigators must ensure that patients in each observational cohort have similar probabilities of being included in each exposure (or treatment) group regardless of demographics and other baseline characteristics. One method of minimizing this risk is using propensity score matching, which is explained in detail in Chap. 13.

Finally, attrition bias (also known as nonresponder bias) is the systematic exclusion of data from a subset of patients whose data is censored due to loss to follow-up. When there is a differential loss to follow-up (e.g., one group has a higher rate of attrition than another), this can introduce bias into data analysis. Non-differential loss to follow-up (e.g., similar rates of loss to follow-up between study groups) is less likely to result in attrition bias, although it is still possible.

To illustrate the possible situations in which selection bias may occur, consider a study that aims to show that a new drug (Drug X) can decrease the 5-year mortality of patients with breast cancer. Investigators plan to enroll a sample of patients with breast cancer, provide Drug X or current standard of care, and follow them for 5 years to calculate differences in 5-year mortality.

- During recruitment, imagine the researchers want to enroll as many participants as possible. They utilize social media platforms in order to engage the largest number of potential participants. This is a source of selection bias as younger patients may be more likely than older patients to use social media. If study samples recruited through social media are younger than the general population of interest, the study results may not be applicable to all patients with that specific cancer diagnosis. Furthermore, if younger age increases the likelihood of Drug X success, this will bias the results away from the null hypothesis and increase the chances of a type I error. The new drug would appear to work better than the current standard of care when, in fact, this may be untrue or only true in younger patients with breast cancer.
- During study group assignment, imagine that the new drug is truly a better medication with improved 5-year survival. However, it is only available at select urban tertiary care cancer specialty hospitals, while the current standard of care medication is available at both specialty and general hospitals. If the only patients receiving the new drug are those at tertiary care specialty hospitals (where perhaps

patients with more aggressive, complex, or later stage disease present referred in from surrounding community hospitals), this would bias results toward the null hypothesis. In this scenario, there are increased chances of a type II error. The new drug would not demonstrate an advantage over the current standard of care when, in fact, it is the superior treatment option. This is due in large part to group imbalance whereby group assignment is inadvertently related to disease severity.

- Finally, during follow-up and data collection, it is possible that patients treated at urban tertiary care cancer specialty hospitals travel farther for care compared to those treated at local hospitals. Those travelling farther distances for care may be more likely to be lost to follow-up than those being treated closer to home, leading to a differential loss to follow-up and attrition bias. Additionally, if patients with more complex or aggressive cancers are potentially cared for at tertiary care cancer specialty hospitals, there may be bias away from the null hypothesis since there will be fewer patients lost to follow-up at local hospitals. This would result in a more accurate 5-year mortality rate in that group. With increased data censoring at the specialty care hospitals, there may be an underestimation of 5-year mortality (as more patients will be lost to follow-up), yielding falsely improved mortality outcomes in the specialty care hospital group.

Incorporation Bias

Incorporation bias is a type of verification bias that occurs when results of a test or variable in question are part of (or incorporated into) the reference test (or gold standard) [1]. This occurs most frequently when the reference test is a composite of the results of several tests.

Incorporation bias is more likely to occur when the gold standard test relies on clinical judgment, which often includes in part the diagnostic test being studied. Incorporation bias will result in an overestimation of the diagnostic test's accuracy. Consider a study that evaluates elevated serum C-reactive protein levels as a predictive test of musculoskeletal infection. The study plans to identify cases of musculoskeletal infection based on judgment by a panel of experts who retrospectively review the medical records. If those records include serum C-reactive protein levels, that result may be incorporated into the judgment by the panel of experts and bias their judgment of whether an infection exists. This would bias the study away from the null hypothesis and, likely, overestimate the predictive value of serum C-reactive protein for predicting musculoskeletal infection.

Financial Bias

Financial bias, also referred to as "funding bias," describes the predisposition of a scientific study to advance the objectives of the study's financial sponsor. Examples include a government agency or a pharmaceutical company that may have an influence on the planning, implementation, analysis, or reporting of a study. When a study is funded by a particular entity, there is a risk that the study findings may be biased in favor of the sponsor's interests and may not be representative of the true effects of the intervention being investigated. For instance, a pharmaceutical company may be more likely to fund studies that are designed to more likely show positive results for their drug but will overlook research that may not support the drug's use.

Perhaps at worst, funding bias can also occur when the sponsor has control over the research question, the selection of study participants, the methodology, the data analysis, or the interpretation of results. Funding sources occasionally have the right to block publication or dissemination of study findings. This can lead to a conflict of interest, where the sponsor's financial interests are prioritized over scientific integrity.

It is important for researchers to disclose their funding sources and potential conflicts of interest to mitigate funding bias. It is best to err on the side of full disclosure. Research institutions and journals should also have rigorous standards for transparency and independence in medical research established to minimize the risk of funding bias. Finally, investigators should ensure that they have full access and rights to any data collected and for publication of their findings, regardless of the study conclusions.

Information Bias

Information bias refers to bias arising from measurement or recording error. Such error can be systematic (consistently in one direction), which can bias results either toward or away from the null hypothesis. The error can also be random, which would result in bias toward the null hypothesis since the direction of error is random and dampens any true association between exposure and outcome. Information bias is also referred to as "observational bias" or "misclassification." Misclassification can be either "differential" or "nondifferential."

Differential Misclassification

Differential misclassification is caused by a measurement difference that exists between study groups, such as a case study group and a control group. Using recall bias as an example, due to heightened awareness and frequent childhood assessments, it is likely that parents of children with cerebral palsy who have developmental delays are able to recall their child's developmental milestones more accurately than parents of typically developing children. They may also be able to recall past exposure to risk factors during pregnancy more accurately than the parents of a healthy control cohort. For that reason, differential misclassification frequently biases results away from the null hypothesis, which overestimates the effect of an exposure (e.g., pregnancy risk factors) on an outcome (e.g., cerebral palsy). However, if the outcome of interest itself can affect memory (e.g., dementia), then it is possible that controls may recall more accurately; hence, differential misclassification can at times also cause an underestimate of the association between predictor variables and outcomes.

Non-differential Misclassification

Non-differential misclassification is caused by inaccurate measurements that affect all study groups to a similar degree. To continue with the recall bias example, it is possible that patients in all study groups have equal difficulty accurately remembering a predictor variable of interest in their history that is not objectively verifiable. Examples include levels of alcohol consumption, precise amount of prior nicotine use, or sun exposure. Because recall bias is similar among all participant groups, there is random error being introduced. This can dampen the magnitude of an existing effect by effectively decreasing the signal to noise ratio. As a result, non-differential misclassification, such as recall bias, tends to exaggerate similarities among study groups. This underestimates any associations being investigated.

Other Types of Information Bias

In addition to recall bias, two additional types of information bias include "observer bias" and "performance bias." Observer bias happens when researchers who are collecting outcome data know to which group a participant is assigned. Such information may influence how researchers collect, measure, or interpret information. Similarly, performance bias refers to situations in which study participants or researchers modify their behavior because they are aware of group allocation. This results in the inadvertent introduction of differences between randomized groups other than the intervention(s) being studied. Such departures from the intended study design may compromise the study and make it challenging to draw valid inferences about intervention effects.

In the case of performance bias, the investigators, study participants, or both can compromise study validity because the observed outcome can be attributed either to the exposure/treatment or to unequal care or behavior between groups. Performance bias alters study results unpredictably, which makes it hard to control in post hoc analyses. It can adversely affect observational studies as well as randomized controlled trials. There is a subtype of performance bias known as the Hawthorne effect where study participants may change their behavior simply because they are aware that they are being studied.

Publication and Reporting Bias

Publication bias occurs when studies with statistically significant findings or hypothesis-affirming results are more likely to be published than those with negative results. This can be driven by investigators (e.g., reporting bias), funding agencies (e.g., funding bias, described above), or peer reviewers (true publication bias). Studies published in peer-reviewed journals are more likely to report statistically significant results than studies that report nonsignificant results [2]. In the absence of publication bias, a well-designed, appropriately powered study would have the same chances of being accepted for publication regardless of the outcome of the study.

When publication bias is present, published studies are no longer a representative sample of the available evidence. In addition to affecting the body of available literature, publication bias skews the outcomes of systematic reviews and meta-analyses, especially when it is not considered or addressed [3, 4]. This is particularly influential as systematic reviews and meta-analyses are becoming increasingly important in evidence-based medicine.

References

1. Worster A, Carpenter C. Incorporation bias in studies of diagnostic tests: how to avoid being biased about bias. CJEM. 2008;10:174–5. https://doi.org/10.1017/s1481803500009891.
2. Hopewell S, Loudon K, Clarke MJ, et al. Publication bias in clinical trials due to statistical significance or direction of trial results. Cochrane Database Syst Rev. 2009; https://doi.org/10.1002/14651858.MR000006.pub3.
3. Marks-Anglin A, Chen Y. A historical review of publication bias. Res synth. Methods. 2020;11:725–42. https://doi.org/10.1002/jrsm.1452.
4. Sutton AJ, Song F, Gilbody SM, et al. Modelling publication bias in meta-analysis: a review. Stat Methods Med Res. 2000;9:421–45. https://doi.org/10.1177/096228020000900503.

Chapter 7
The Iterative Process of Designing Successful Clinical Research

Introduction

Effectively formulating a research question is the first and perhaps most important step in designing a successful study. Doing so requires a careful and systematic process, beginning with a comprehensive literature search to understand existing literature and gaps in knowledge. Conversely, an incomplete knowledge of existing literature could result in a large time investment toward conducting a study that has already been done or may not meaningfully contribute to current knowledge.

Research questions should be formulated precisely and with operationalized variables that are measurable, valid, and clinically meaningful. Operationalization is the process of defining abstract concepts though measurable observations and quantifiably defining variables to make them useful for clinical research [1]. Graphical depiction of a proposed study using directed acyclic graphs (DAGs) can be effective at depicting hypothesized relationships and framing an operationalized research question. Finally, prior to patient enrollment or data collection, the feasibility of completion and publication of a proposed study is important to consider at the outset. Regularly scheduled meetings with mentors and peers will facilitate the study's progress and minimize the risk of regrettable oversights with data collection and analysis.

Formulating a Study Question

When formulating a study question, it is important to be as precise and specific as possible. Frequently, research questions begin as conversations, which are vague but stimulate ideas for research. It is the duty of the researcher to craft that conversational idea into a study question.

For example, a conversation might start with, "We should take a look at how our patients who undergo anterior cruciate ligament (ACL) reconstruction do

© The Author(s), under exclusive license to Springer Nature Switzerland AG 2024
P. D. Fabricant, *Practical Clinical Research Design and Application*,
https://doi.org/10.1007/978-3-031-58380-3_7

postoperatively." This is an important idea but has not been formulated into a precise research question. Getting more specific, this could be refined to, "We should investigate which ACL graft is better, graft A or graft B." While this is more specific, it does not identify a study population in whom this question is pressing or important. It can be further revised to "We should investigate which ACL graft is better, graft A or graft B, in adolescent female soccer players." This now becomes a more precise research question, as adolescent female soccer players tend to have the greatest risk of subsequent ACL reinjury and graft tear. A final iteration of this research question could specify in detail, "We should investigate which ACL graft is better, graft A or graft B, in adolescent female soccer players 14-18 years old, as measured by rate of re-rupture in the first 5 years postoperatively."

In this way, one hones an important research question which is focused, precise, and with an operationalized outcome. A mnemonic to consider when formulating a research question is PICO. Give careful consideration to each of the following:

- **P**atient, Population, or Problem
- **I**ntervention
- **C**omparison
- **O**utcome

Operationalizing Variables

"Operationalizing" variables is the process of precisely defining what will be measured and is a vital component to formulating a research question. The example above, "which ACL graft is better," was operationalized to "which ACL graft is better… as measured by rate of re-rupture in the first 5 years postoperatively." By operationalizing the study variables, it encourages the researcher to consider more precisely what outcomes are most important.

When choosing variables to measure, the researcher must choose variables that are:

1. *Measurable and Quantifiable*: Variables (both dependent and independent) must be measurable and quantifiable to be analyzed.
2. *Valid/Validated in the Cohort of Interest*: Particularly with patient reported outcome measures (PROMs), it is important to choose outcomes that are valid for the clinical condition being investigated in the study population of interest (e.g., pediatric-specific questionnaires for young athletes). This ensures that those outcome measures are appropriate and applicable to those patients. Alternatively, hard outcomes (typically binary, e.g., death, infection, reinjury, treatment failure) are usually not specially validated in a cohort or condition of interest, but nonetheless are clinically meaningful.
3. *Meaningful*: For an outcome measure to be acceptable to the scientific or medical community at large, it is important that it is clinically meaningful. If the authors of a study argue in favor of changing practice, they must improve outcomes that clinicians, researchers, and patients believe to be important. This should be considered when designing any clinical research study.

Directed Acyclic Graphs (DAGs)

By constructing directed acyclic graphs (DAGs) researchers can graphically depict hypothesized relationships and the possible effects of covariables. DAGs further help investigators deduce the statistical associations implied by these relationships and help frame a detailed and operationalized research question.

To start, one can map out the main hypothesized effect, "X causes Y." Then, consider if "Y" could also cause "X," determine if "X" and "Y" have a common cause, and what other variables may be associated with "X," "Y," and other common causes. To do this, one would start with the exposure-outcome relationship, next add in all common causes of exposure and outcome, and finally enter all common causes of all the variables. As their name would imply, DAGs must be acyclical, meaning that no variable can cause (or be) its own cause.

The most frequent components of DAGs are noted in Fig. 7.1 and include main effect, confounders, mediators, and effect measure modifiers (i.e., interactions).

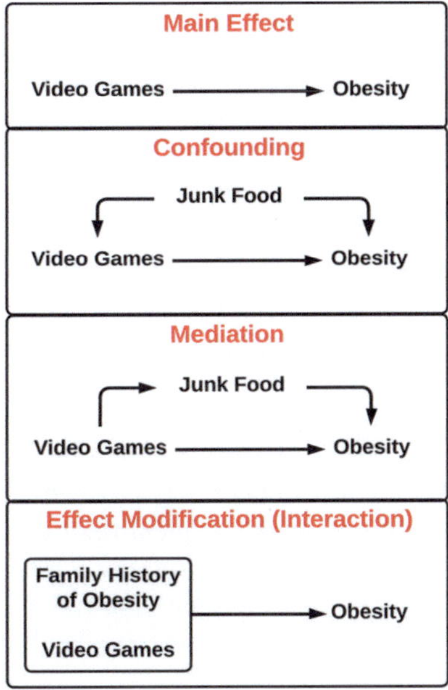

Fig. 7.1 Use of DAGs is illustrated in the following example. The main effect being investigated is that exposure to excessive video game play is associated with obesity. Then the investigator can consider confounding and mediation. Whether a variable is a confounder or mediator is based on whether the variable in question is simply associated with both the exposure and outcome (i.e., confounding) or the variable is the result of the exposure (in this case, that playing video games leads to increased junk food consumption, which in turn causes obesity). Statistically, a confounding or mediating variable (in this case, consumption of junk food) must both be significantly associated with both the outcome and main explanatory variable, and controlling for that variable in regression analysis changes the magnitude of the main effect by 10% or greater. Finally, effect modification (also known as interaction) occurs when an independent variable has a different effect on the outcome depending on another (and sometimes unrelated) independent variable. In this example, the combination of family history of obesity and excessive video game play has a synergistic effect on the risk of developing obesity. Neither of the two might have as a dramatic effect individually

Feasibility

An early feasibility assessment is paramount to any research study. In the process of designing a study, a researcher must consider whether the study can be performed and completed with respect to timeline, eligible patient quantity, and if the available resources are sufficient (time, funds, space, infrastructure, support). If not, then one must consider adjusting the research strategy, increasing the resources available, or both.

Furthermore, prior to initiating the study, one must consider the implications of positive or negative study results. In many instances, a positive study (perhaps one that could change practice) may be more likely to be published and have an impact than a negative study [2]. But in some instances, a study may have difficulty finding acceptance regardless of a positive or negative result. This may be the case where a proposed intervention may be shown to be beneficial in the research setting but is impractical in the clinical setting (e.g., too expensive, too drastic, or requires overly specialized infrastructure). In such a situation, if a study is unlikely to be impactful regardless of the outcome, it should be reconsidered. Conversely, some studies are of interest whether the results are positive or negative. This is the ideal kind of study, as the chances of creating a meaningful contribution to existing knowledge does not rely on the outcome of the investigation.

Peer and Mentor Review

In this final phase of study design, the researcher seeks out peers, colleagues, and mentors who can serve to constructively challenge the research idea, plan, and justification. These partners force the investigator to consider additional or related ideas to incorporate into the study. They can pose the "what if…" questions that are vital to consider at the study design phase, when improvements can be made before the study starts. Otherwise, the investigator may proceed with a flawed study which may not be exposed until a journal reviewer identifies the same concern that would be impossible to address after study completion. Early identification and correction of study design flaws and weaknesses mitigate the risk of diminished impact and validity during later phases of manuscript production and publication.

The Iterative Process

After each of the above processes, the final step is to consider revisions and improvements to each of the components (Fig. 7.2). As each step is revised, additional modifications may be necessary in other parts. By going through several iterations of revision, the study design will become more precise and refined, which improves the chance of successful completion.

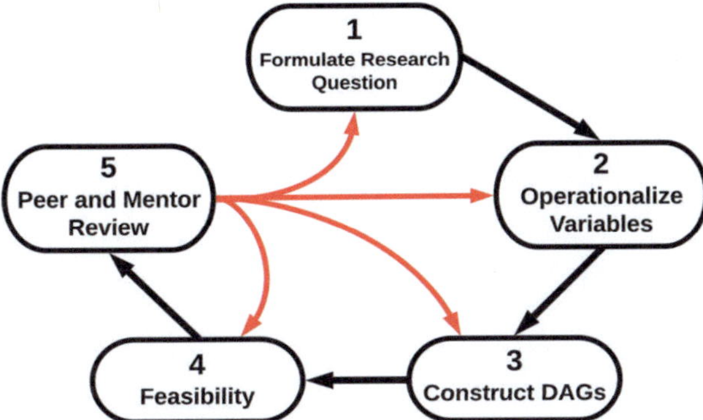

Fig. 7.2 Designing successful clinical research requires an iterative process. After moving through each step, engaging colleagues and mentors for review improves each facet of the study. With each iteration, the study design will become more precise and refined, which results in an increased chance of successful completion. DAGs: directed acyclic graphs

References

1. Heath C. What is operationalization? Dovetail Research Pty. Ltd.; 2023. https://dovetail.com/research/operationalization/. Accessed 18 Dec 2023.
2. Hopewell S, Loudon K, Clarke MJ, et al. Publication bias in clinical trials due to statistical significance or direction of trial results. Cochrane Database Syst Rev. 2009; https://doi.org/10.1002/14651858.MR000006.pub3.

Part II
Choosing and Executing an Appropriate
Clinical Study Design

Chapter 8
Randomized Controlled Trials

Randomized controlled trials	
Pros	Cons
Level 1 studies (highest level of clinical evidence)	Expensive to conduct
Greatest impact on clinical care	Time consuming
	Need robust operational and regulatory structure to perform

Study Mechanics

Prospective randomized controlled trials (RCTs) represent the highest level of evidence available in medical literature. They are unique from other study designs (e.g., case-control studies, cross-sectional studies, cohort studies, case series) in that they are experimental rather than observational. RCTs are performed to compare the effects of drugs, devices, diagnostic procedures, surgeries, or other treatments which are assigned and experimentally controlled by the investigator, rather than simply observed (Fig. 8.1).

Several criteria must be met to determine whether an RCT is an appropriate investigational strategy. First, there must be clinical equipoise (e.g., there is not one treatment with clear superiority). There must also be sufficient existing observational data to support the need for an RCT. Randomized trials are not the first line of study for a clinical question, but in some cases, the experimental study design is required to build upon existing observational data and determine an optimal intervention. Finally, the use of placebo treatment is ethically justifiable when there are no existing standard treatments or as long as patients will not be harmed (e.g., postponement of treatment for duration of patient data collection would unlikely alter the disease course).

P. D. Fabricant, *Practical Clinical Research Design and Application*, https://doi.org/10.1007/978-3-031-58380-3_8

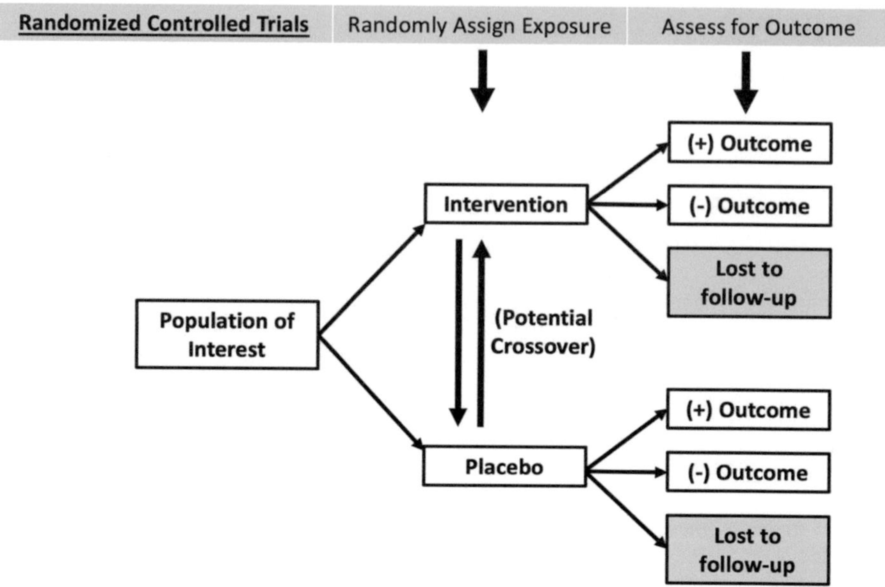

Fig. 8.1 Flow of study participants through a randomized controlled trial

RCTs are employed in Phase III of U.S. Food and Drug Administration (FDA) sanctioned clinical trials when a new drug or device is brought to market in the United States. During the clinical trial process, phase I evaluates the safety of a drug in a small group of unaffected individuals. Phase II evaluates safety, dosing (in the case of drugs), and efficacy in a slightly larger group of affected individuals. In phase III, prospective RCTs are used to demonstrate superiority (or non-inferiority) of the study treatment compared to a control or comparison group. After approval, phase IV is composed of post-marketing surveillance to monitor for any long-term or rare complications or adverse effects.

When designing RCTs, there are three frequently used methods for group allocation:

- *Parallel group*: Parallel group design is the most straightforward and common RCT study design. In a parallel group study design, each participant is randomly assigned to an intervention group. One group receives the intervention of interest, and the other group(s) receive either an alternative intervention (e.g., existing standard of care) or placebo treatment.
- *Crossover*: Crossover study design is the most rigorous study design within RCTs. Each study participant serves as his/her own internal control. However, the interventions and outcomes being studied must meet a list of additional requirements. Specifically, the onset and termination (washout) of the effect of the treatment on the outcome of interest must be rapid. This allows for the measurement of the outcome of interest, a washout period, and alternative intervention. Consider, for example, a new oral blood pressure medication that reaches maximum effectiveness in 1 week. An investigator could assess baseline blood

pressure, then randomly assign each participant to receive the medication or placebo for 2 weeks. Blood pressure response could be measured. Then, study participants could discontinue the first intervention for 2 weeks (to allow for washout of treatment effect). Next, they would get treatment with the alternate intervention for 2 weeks and have blood pressure response measured again. The blood pressure response to each treatment would be compared within each individual participant and across groups.

- *Cluster*: In a cluster study design, pre-existing groups are randomized *en masse* to receive an intervention or placebo treatment. Examples include all patients of one clinic, where all patients in that clinic receive the same intervention or placebo treatment. In such a scenario, each clinic would be randomly assigned to a treatment group and all patients of that clinic would receive the same treatment.

In RCTs, there are three main ways to perform randomization:

- *Simple randomization*: In simple randomization, each study participant is randomly assigned to the intervention or control group. This is ideal for large RCTs and, in that setting, is an effective measure against selection bias. However, in smaller RCTs (e.g., less than 200 participants), this can still lead to imbalanced group sizes or distribution of potential confounding variables due to chance.
- *Restricted randomization*: In restricted randomization, blocks of study participants are identified and randomized within each block. This can include blocks based upon number of participants (e.g., blocks of 10 enrollees) or within stratifications based on a known potential confounder. This way the investigator increases the chances of an equal distribution of a key confounder among study groups. Restricted randomization strategies are required for smaller RCTs. In a large enough study, simple randomization would naturally balance such variables among groups.
- *Adaptive randomization*: This is a less common randomization strategy in which the probability of being assigned to a group will vary based on the development of any covariate imbalances. For example, if during the randomization process, there are more males than females in group A than group B, then a subsequent male participant would more likely be assigned to group B while a subsequent female participant would more likely be assigned to group A. This would proceed until the groups became balanced and the randomization for both males and females would again be 50/50 for each group. Importantly, interim distributions would have to be monitored by an independent reviewer or research staff other than the principal investigator, especially when blinding is being applied.

In RCTs, methodological rigor can be further enhanced by performing a process of allocation concealment (e.g., blinding). Depending on the type of study, any or all of the following parties can be blinded:

- Patients/participants
- Treating clinician(s)
- Study team member(s) measuring or collecting treatment outcomes
- Study team member(s) performing statistical analyses

The more individuals that can be blinded, the more rigorous the study. It is therefore important when designing an RCT to attempt blinding as many of the investigators (and participants) as possible to the group assignment. RCTs in which the administered medication may be unknown to both the treating clinician and the patient are the easiest to blind, while those involving surgery, procedures, and/or new implants are the hardest to blind. Though the study team member who performs the statistical analyses can almost always be blinded, there are some scenarios in which the treating clinician and/or the study participant cannot be blinded. In such cases, potential for bias can be mitigated by implementing non-treating blinded study team members who measure/collect the outcome(s) of interest separately from those who perform data analysis. This is true even in the case of surgical procedures where surgical scars can be obscured from the study team member performing data collection.

- *Examples in which the treating clinician cannot be blinded*:

  - RCTs that compare one procedure, surgical technique, or implant to another (the surgeon or proceduralist must know the procedure being performed)
  - RCTs that compare a surgery or procedure to a non-operative treatment strategy

- *Example in which the study participant cannot be blinded*:

  - RCTs that compare a surgery or procedure to a non-operative treatment strategy

- *Example in which the individual collecting data cannot be blinded*:

  - RCTs that utilize a radiographic outcome in which the treatment is evident in the imaging being analyzed (e.g., an implant that is radiographically distinguishable)

Finally, each prospective RCT should be under the scrutiny of an unblinded data safety monitoring board (DSMB) which independently and regularly monitors the data outside of the purview of the study investigators. The DSMB has the authority to stop an RCT early if either:

- There is an imbalanced frequency of complications in one of the treatment groups, and the DSMB deems it unethical to proceed with continued randomization. One example may be unacceptably higher rates of deep vein thrombosis as a side effect of a study medication. This would justify stopping an RCT early.
- There is an overwhelmingly positive response to the treatment of interest, and the DSMB deems it unethical to proceed with continued randomization. One example may be overwhelming success of a new chemotherapy regimen when compared to an existing standard of care. This would justify stopping the trial early in order to submit data to the FDA to consider approving the study regimen for clinical use.

Ideal Scenario for Prospective Randomized Controlled Trial Study Design

The ideal scenario for an RCT is one in which clinical equipoise exists with a new or alternative treatment available for investigation. Also, the use of placebo, if chosen, should be ethically justifiable. Additionally, study participants, treating clinicians, data collection personnel, and data analysis team should ideally be able to be blinded. In order to have sufficient power, the disease or outcome of interest should be common enough to facilitate adequate enrollment. Finally, in an ideal RCT, the primary outcome of interest is one that does not require long-term follow-up. This minimizes loss to follow-up and cost associated with study procedures.

Statistical Analysis

When preparing to perform an RCT, the investigator must perform a power analysis to determine the number of study participants required to enroll. The components and mechanics of statistical power and power calculations are discussed in detail in Chap. 4.

When analyzing results from an RCT, statistical analysis is typically straightforward. A randomized study design with a sufficiently large cohort creates an equal distribution of variables among groups aside from the intervention of interest. This often eliminates the need to control for covariables with regression analyses. Instead, after confirmation of equal distribution of potential covariables of interest between groups and testing for data normality, the investigator may perform typical analyses described in Chaps. 1, 2, and 3 such as:

- Unpaired Student's t-tests for continuous outcome(s) in two groups
- ANOVA for continuous outcome(s) in 3+ groups
- z-test for proportions
- Chi-squared tests for categorial outcomes

Finally, it is important for investigators to have a plan for dealing with patients who cross over between groups and end up receiving a treatment that they were not originally assigned at randomization. High rates of crossover can undermine the rigor of an RCT, particularly if there is imbalanced crossover (e.g., unidirectional). Crossover can also be problematic when there is an association between crossover and a potential confounding variable, and treatment groups do not have an equal distribution of a potential confounder. The two methods of data analysis to account for crossover are as follows:

- *Intention-to-treat analysis*: Intention-to-treat analysis is typically performed in the setting of medical interventions or those in which patients administer their own treatment. For example, in the setting of an oral medication being investigated where there is a side effect in a subset of patients, there may be unequal crossover because patients assigned to the treatment medication are less compliant than those in the placebo group. In such a scenario, some of the treatment group patients are effectively receiving no medication, which is similar to receiving placebo (those patients inadvertently crossed over from treatment group to placebo group). Because this could wash out a potential treatment effect, it is important to analyze study participants on the basis of the group to which they were randomly assigned, regardless of whether they actually received the medication. This analysis strategy represents a "real world" effect of prescribing that medication to a group of patients. It also provides information about the potential effects of a treatment strategy.

- *As-treated analysis*: Conversely, as-treated analyses are performed based on which study participants actually receive the intended treatment. This is most frequently implemented in surgical or procedural interventions. Patients can cross over into the procedural treatment (e.g., they no longer want non-procedural intervention and elect to receive the procedure) or out of the procedural treatment (e.g., they are assigned the procedure but then decide not to have it). As-treated analyses are used so that the benefits and drawbacks of the treatment are assigned only to those participants who received the treatment, not the treatment they were supposed to receive. Also, noncompliance unbeknownst to the investigators (as was the case in the above intention-to-treat example) is not as problematic in the setting of a procedural interventions.

Analytical Review

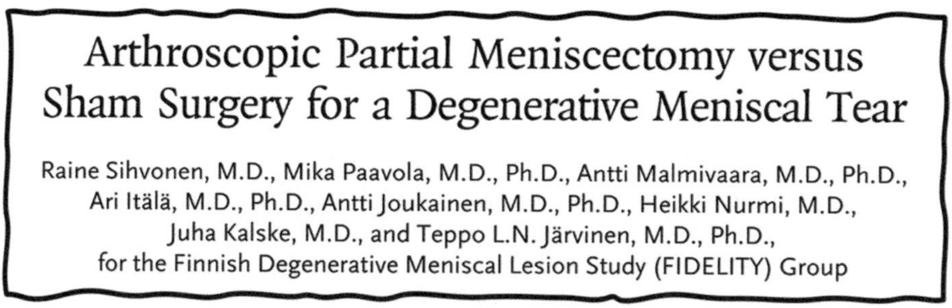

Arthroscopic Partial Meniscectomy versus Sham Surgery for a Degenerative Meniscal Tear

Raine Sihvonen, M.D., Mika Paavola, M.D., Ph.D., Antti Malmivaara, M.D., Ph.D., Ari Itälä, M.D., Ph.D., Antti Joukainen, M.D., Ph.D., Heikki Nurmi, M.D., Juha Kalske, M.D., and Teppo L.N. Järvinen, M.D., Ph.D., for the Finnish Degenerative Meniscal Lesion Study (FIDELITY) Group

Fig. 8.2 Illustrative example of a prospective randomized controlled trial by Sihvonen R, et al. [1]

An example of a surgical prospective RCT study is illustrated in (Fig. 8.2).

In their 2013 RCT, Sihvonen and colleagues investigated the effectiveness of arthroscopic partial meniscectomy, the most common orthopedic procedure in the United States at the time [1]. Their multicenter prospective RCT, led by the Finnish Degenerative Meniscal Lesion Study (FIDELITY) group, enrolled patients between the ages of 35 and 65 years old who had knee symptoms consistent with a degenerative medial meniscus tear and no knee osteoarthritis. Although arthroscopic partial meniscectomy was the most common orthopedic procedure at the time, it was unclear what effect the procedure had beyond other treatment modalities, such as physical therapy, on alleviating symptoms of degenerative meniscal tears.

After a potentially eligible patient provided informed consent, the surgeon performed diagnostic arthroscopic surgery to confirm the presence of a degenerative meniscal tear. Intraoperatively, an envelope was opened to disclose the randomized intervention which the patient would receive either an arthroscopic partial meniscectomy or sham surgery. In order to minimize differences in the treatment arms, the randomization occurred after the initial diagnostic arthroscopy. Those who received the sham surgery were kept in the operating room and the knee was brought through similar maneuvers (albeit without performing the actual meniscectomy).

The primary outcomes of interest were the Lysholm and WOMET scores (validated, knee-specific patient-reported outcome measures) and knee pain after exercise at 12 months postoperatively. An a priori power analysis using existing data from a previous prospective cohort study by the same group determined that 70 participants would be needed in each group to detect clinically relevant differences in Lysholm and WOMET scores. One hundred and forty-six patients were enrolled to minimize the risk of type II error (e.g., to adequately power the study). While it was impossible to blind the surgeon to the treatment provided, neither the patient nor the clinician performing the follow-up were aware of the intervention. Because the incisions are the same for both interventions, the visual appearance of the knee at follow-up is identical. Neither patients nor clinicians could determine the treatment based on the visual appearance of the knee. The investigators found no differences in any of the outcomes analyzed. Therefore, they concluded that arthroscopic partial meniscectomy was not superior to sham surgery (in essence, nonsurgical treatment) for patients with degenerative medial meniscus tears in the absence of knee osteoarthritis.

A double-blinded RCT (blinding both the patient and data collector) is an ideal study design to answer this clinical question. It eliminates the potential for selection bias and blinds the study participants and investigators collecting follow-up data from the procedure that was performed. There can be a substantial "placebo effect" for a study of surgical versus nonsurgical treatment. After surgery, a patient may feel as though a thorough intervention was performed, and as a result, may invest more time and effort in postoperative physical therapy than a patient being treated with physical therapy alone. However, in this study, the potential for placebo effect is eliminated because both groups received an identical arthroscopic surgery (with the exception of the meniscectomy) and postoperative treatment. Furthermore, the randomization and assigned treatment happened in the same setting, so the risk of crossover was also eliminated. Finally, the multicenter nature of this investigation increases generalizability of the findings. These strengths contributed to this investigation's designation as a landmark study that changed clinical practice. Arthroscopic partial meniscectomies are now recommended for the treatment of patients with mechanical symptoms (such as knee locking) rather than for knee pain in isolation.

Reference

1. Sihvonen R, Paavola M, Malmivaara A, et al. Arthroscopic partial meniscectomy versus sham surgery for a degenerative meniscal tear. N Engl J Med. 2013;369:2515–24. https://doi.org/10.1056/NEJMoa1305189.

Chapter 9
Case-Control Studies

Case-control studies	
Pros	Cons
No loss to follow-up because outcome has already happened (or not)	Subject to recall bias (if exposure is not documented and requires participant to remember details about exposure)
Ideal for rare outcomes; oversampling of patients with the rare outcome gives more balanced comparison groups	Requires large sample size if exposure is rare
Given appropriate dataset, retrospective study design is fast and inexpensive	

Study Mechanics

Case-control studies are unique in that cases and controls are *sampled based on the presence or absence of an outcome*. Then patients are compared to see if they had previously experienced the exposure(s) of interest. This is different from a comparative cohort study where a cohort is classified based on if it experienced an exposure (independent variable). Then the cohort is queried on an outcome (dependent variable). This definition is true regardless of whether or not patients are matched on other covariables (Fig. 9.1).

A case-control design provides several distinct advantages over cohort studies:

- There is no censoring (e.g., loss to follow-up) or unknown outcome status. Unlike comparative cohort studies, outcome is known from the beginning in a case-control study. It is the variable upon which cases and controls are selected.
- In a cohort study, a large sample size is required in order to accumulate enough outcome events to power an analysis when an outcome is rare. However, in a case-control study, oversampling of patients with the rare outcome gives more balanced groups.

P. D. Fabricant, *Practical Clinical Research Design and Application*, https://doi.org/10.1007/978-3-031-58380-3_9

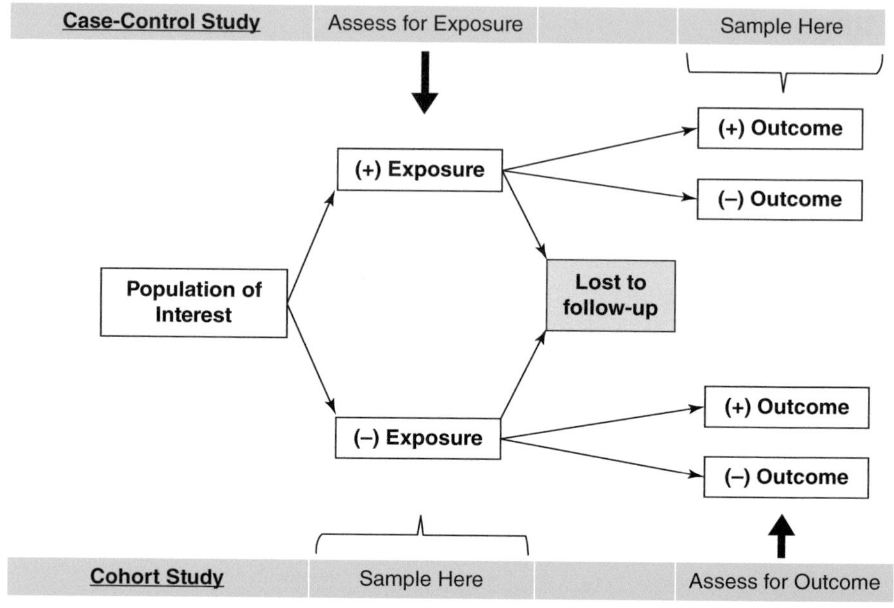

Fig. 9.1 Sampling and analysis frameworks are opposite for case-control and cohort studies. In case-control studies (top), patients are sampled based on the outcome, and then the investigator assesses for the exposure of interest. In cohort studies (bottom), patients are sampled based on exposure, and then the investigator assesses for the outcome of interest

Despite these strengths, the main limitation of a case-control study is the potential for recall bias because patients are required to recall if they experienced the exposure of interest. Recall bias can be minimized if the exposure of interest is one that is life-altering or traumatic (e.g., a fracture, trauma, etc.), involves an exposure as part of a daily routine (e.g., smoking, coffee consumption, etc.), or is documented in the medical record (e.g., medication given by a physician).

Ideal Scenario for Case-Control Study Design

The ideal scenario for a case-control design is when there is a large population of interest but the outcome or disease in question is rare. Additionally, if the exposure is difficult or expensive to measure (e.g., requires a challenging lab test or tissue sample), a case-control design allows the investigator to focus on a smaller study cohort. This ensures an adequate number of positive outcomes (which may also be rare in the larger population). This way, resources dedicated to measuring the exposure of interest can focus on a subset of patients, rather than on a much larger cohort, which would be required to accumulate the number of rare outcomes in sufficient quantity to adequately power the study.

	Outcome or Disease (+) [Cases]	Outcome or Disease (–) [Controls]
Exposure (+)	A	B
Exposure (–)	C	D

$$OR = \frac{\text{odds of exposure given outcome or disease}}{\text{odds of exposure given no outcome or disease}} = \frac{A/C}{B/D}$$

Fig. 9.2 Odds ratio for a case-control study is the odds of exposure in the cases (A/C) divided by the odds of exposure in the controls (B/D)

Statistical Analysis

When performing statistical analysis for a case-control study, it is important to remember that patients are selected based on whether or not they have the outcome of interest (rather than exposure). Because the incidence of the outcome of interest is artificially set by the investigator, risk ratios should not be used. In other words, if the true incidence of a rare disease or outcome is 0.1% of the population, but the investigator constructs a case-control study with a 1:3 match, then the incidence of the outcome in the study population would be incorrectly assigned as 25% of the study cohort. Similarly, if the study is constructed with a 1:1 match, the incidence of the outcome in the study population is 50%.

In both scenarios, the incidence of the disease or outcome is completely controlled by the investigator constructing the study. Therefore, the rate and risk ratios (e.g., the risk of developing the disease/outcome) are not meaningful. Instead, odds ratios are utilized to communicate the odds of having experienced the exposure of interest given the outcome of interest (Fig. 9.2).

Analytical Review

Development of arthrosis following dislocation of the shoulder: A case-control study

Robert G. Marx, MD, MSc, FRCS(C), Eric C. McCarty, MD, T. Deborah Montemurno, BS, David W. Altchek, MD, Edward V. Craig, MD, and Russell F. Warren, MD

Fig. 9.3 Illustrative example of a case-control study by Marx RG, et al. [1]

An example of a case-control study is illustrated in (Fig. 9.3).

In their 2002 study, Marx and colleagues utilized a case-control study design to investigate for a relationship between a history of glenohumeral (shoulder) dislocation and glenohumeral arthritis requiring shoulder arthroplasty (replacement) [1]. The authors identified patients with osteoarthritis who had undergone total or partial shoulder arthroplasty as *cases* to perform this study. This ideal cohort with severe disease (requiring surgical intervention) was easily identifiable because the diagnosis could be confirmed at surgery. Controls consisted of patients who had undergone total knee arthroplasty, as a similar group who had arthritis in a different joint. Both groups were asked about a history of previous shoulder dislocation. Controls were also asked about pain, stiffness, trouble with activities of daily living, and previous surgery or injections in their shoulder to exclude those with any possibility of clinically relevant shoulder arthrosis from the control group.

The investigators calculated the odds of having sustained a shoulder dislocation for each group, and then calculated the odds ratio from a standard 2×2 table:

	Shoulder arthritis (+) requiring shoulder arthroplasty [cases]	Shoulder arthritis (−) knee arthroplasty patients [controls]
History of shoulder dislocation	11	2
No history of shoulder dislocation	80	280

$$OR = \frac{11/80}{2/280} = \frac{0.1375}{0.0071} = 19.3$$

The authors concluded: Patients with advanced shoulder arthritis undergoing shoulder arthroplasty had 19.3 times greater odds of having sustained a previous shoulder dislocation compared to controls.

This clinical question was ideal for a case-control study design for the following reasons:

- Prevalence of shoulder arthritis requiring arthroplasty is rare. At the time of publication, it was noted to be <1% of the population.
- Similarly, shoulder dislocations are rare events. At the time, epidemiologic studies noted occurrences affected between 0.5% and 1.7% of the population.
- The duration from glenohumeral dislocation to the development of shoulder arthritis takes many years, which would require extensive follow-up and, consequently, excessive resources.

In order to perform a similar investigation prospectively, the authors would have to track a large cohort of patients for a prolonged period. This would be expensive, impractical, and likely lead to incomplete data from loss to follow-up. By performing a case-control study, the authors were able to focus on a smaller cohort with a known outcome (presence or absence of shoulder arthritis). They identified an appropriate control group of total knee arthroplasty controls (who were of similar age and health as the shoulder arthroplasty cases). Finally, with a longer time interval between exposure and outcome, recall bias is often a concern in case-control studies. However, the authors identified an exposure which is less likely to be subject to recall bias: anyone who dislocates a shoulder requiring a reduction is unlikely to forget that experience.

Reference

1. Marx RG, McCarty EC, Montemurno TD, et al. Development of arthrosis following dislocation of the shoulder: a case-control study. J Shoulder Elbow Surg. 2002;11:1–5. https://doi.org/10.1067/mse.2002.119388.

Chapter 10
Cohort Studies

Cohort studies	
Pros	Cons
Can quantify a temporal relationship between exposure and outcome	Requires longitudinal follow-up or detailed records to quantify outcomes
Ideal for rare exposures	Requires large sample size if disease or outcome is rare
Prospective cohort studies are not subject to recall bias	Subject to loss to follow-up; can lead to biased results if uneven between groups
Retrospective cohort studies are fast, easy, and inexpensive to perform	Prospective cohort studies can be expensive, especially with larger cohorts that require long-term follow-up

Study Mechanics

Cohort studies are prospective or retrospective observational studies in which groups of study participants are identified and classified based on exposure. The exposure of interest can be a specific disease, treatment, or both. Then, participants in each group are assessed for outcomes and compared. Although there are single cohort investigations (e.g., without a comparison cohort), these differ from case series only in the number of participants enrolled. Journals set various thresholds for the number of participants needed to constitute a cohort study rather than a smaller case series. For the purposes of this chapter, only comparative cohort studies with ≥2 groups will be discussed.

It is critical to distinguish a cohort study with a comparison or control group from a case-control study. The cohort study design differs from case-control study design in that the cohort is generated from a population of interest based on the exposure. Then participants are compared on the basis of their outcome of interest (Fig. 10.1). Although they may seem similar at first, these differences impact statistical analyses and how results are reported.

© The Author(s), under exclusive license to Springer Nature
Switzerland AG 2024

P. D. Fabricant, *Practical Clinical Research Design and Application*,
https://doi.org/10.1007/978-3-031-58380-3_10

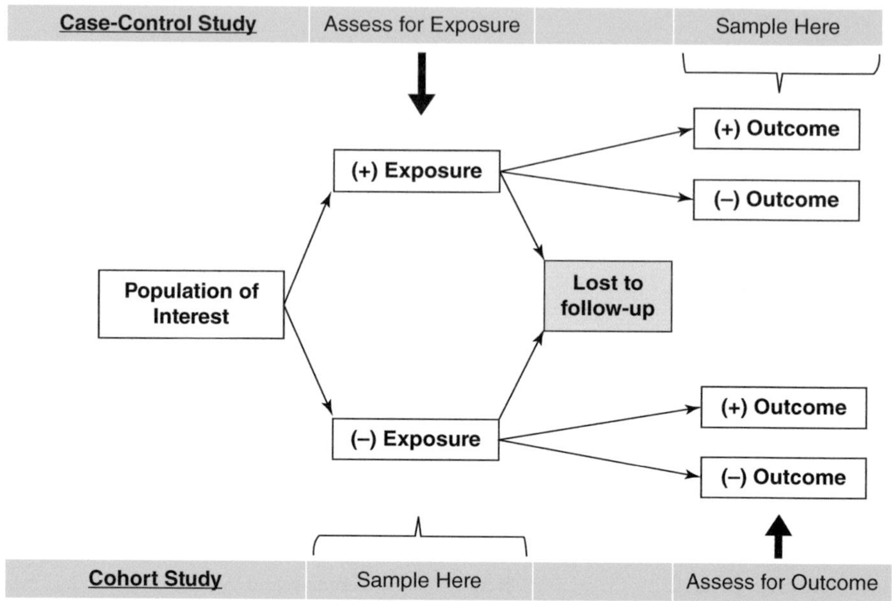

Fig. 10.1 Sampling and analysis frameworks are opposite for case-control and cohort studies. In case-control studies (top), patients are sampled based on the outcome and then assessed for the exposure of interest. In cohort studies (bottom), patients are sampled based on the exposure and then the investigator assesses for the outcome of interest

For example, if one were to design a study testing the association between smoking and developing cancer:

- A prospective *cohort study* would enroll smokers and non-smokers and follow them prospectively to assess the difference in the risk of developing cancer using a risk ratio or odds ratio.
- A *case-control study* would enroll patients with and without cancer (cases and controls, respectively) matched on covariables of interest, then investigate the odds of prior exposure to smoking in each group. Only an odds ratio can be reported (further explained in Chap. 9).

There are advantages to the cohort study design:

- Unlike case-control studies, prospective cohort studies are not subject to recall bias because patients are identified and stratified based on exposure and then followed for the outcome of interest.
- Because patients have not experienced the outcome of interest at the time of exposure and the study is longitudinal, the time between exposure and outcome can be measured.
- Provided existing data is high-quality, retrospective cohort studies are fast, easy, and inexpensive compared to other study types that can only be performed prospectively.

Despite these advantages, drawbacks of the cohort study design include:

- Prospective cohort studies are subject to loss to follow-up. Differential loss to follow-up or data censoring can lead to biased results.
- When an outcome is rare, a large sample size is required to accumulate enough outcome events to power an analysis.
- Prospective cohort studies can be expensive, especially with larger cohorts that require long-term follow-up.

Ideal Scenario for Cohort Study Design

The ideal scenario for a cohort study design is when there is a large population from which to draw a cohort of interest, a short timeframe from exposure to outcome, and the outcome is not exceedingly rare. In this situation, it would not be difficult to identify (and for a prospective study design, enroll) patients. Additionally, the short follow-up interval would minimize costs of following patients and the problems arising from losing them to follow-up.

Consider the association between sex and 90-day mortality after myocardial infarction being investigated at a large academic cardiac center. There would be a large population from which to enroll participants, the exposure of interest (in this case sex) is easily measurable, and 90-day follow-up is sufficiently short to minimize the risk of loss to follow-up. Similarly, minimal resources would be required to complete such a study due to both the short follow-up interval and the simplicity of the outcome measurement (90-day mortality). Alternatively, investigating a rarer condition using an outcome that is more challenging to measure (i.e., ejection fraction using echocardiogram) and/or with long-term follow-up would require more resources in order to complete a cohort study investigating a similar question.

Cohort Study Patient Selection

There are several important factors related to cohort selection during study design that must be considered. Inclusion and exclusion criteria are important to delineate at the outset to answer the study question and allow for generalizability. In the case of a comparative cohort study, an a priori power calculation should be performed to ensure there will be sufficient patients and minimize the risk of type II error (Chap. 4).

Cohort studies are most often affected by selection bias (Chap. 6). It is important to consider this possibility when designing both retrospective and prospective cohort studies. In a retrospective cohort study, selection from available patients with sufficient follow-up to measure the clinical outcome of interest may result in deceptively positive outcomes. Those who had complications of treatment may have sought further care elsewhere, thus records may not be available. One method to mitigate this possibility is to compare the length of follow-up of those who are included and analyzed to those who were excluded to ensure they are no different. Similarly, in prospective cohort studies, loss to follow-up can be a significant concern. In a comparative cohort study design, differential loss to follow-up between groups can lead to biased results. Other sources of selection bias can also be problematic for retrospective cohort studies with short-term follow-up. These include missing data or incorrect diagnosis coding in medical record reviews.

One method to limit confounding in comparative cohort studies is to control for potential confounders during statistical analyses or match patients between exposure groups based on similar confounders (e.g., demographic variables, clinical variables, length of follow-up, etc.).

Statistical Analysis

Statistical analysis for a cohort study may be simple or complex depending on the study cohort and outcome(s) being evaluated.

While case-control studies must report odds ratios because cases and controls are selected based on the outcome of interest (Chap. 9), cohort studies may report odds ratios or risk ratios because they are designed based on the exposure or disease of interest. Relative risk (i.e., risk ratios) and attributable risk (i.e., risk difference) are calculated as illustrated in Fig. 10.2.

	Outcome/Event (+)	Outcome/Event (-)
Exposure (+)	A	B
Exposure (-)	C	D

$$\text{Relative Risk} = \frac{\textit{Incidence Risk (Exposed)}}{\textit{Incidence Risk (Unexposed)}} = \frac{A/(A+B)}{C/(C+D)}$$

$$\text{Attributable Risk} = \textit{Incidence Risk (Exposed)} - \textit{Incidence Risk (Unexposed)}$$

$$= \frac{A}{A+B} - \frac{C}{C+D}$$

Fig. 10.2 Relative risk (i.e., risk ratio) is how many times greater the risk of an outcome is given the exposure of interest. Attributable risk (i.e., risk difference) is the proportion of an outcome in exposed patients that can be attributed to the exposure. Calculating both values can be helpful in communicating study results. For example, if the risk of an outcome in exposed patients is 4 in 10,000 but in unexposed patients is 1 in 10,000, the relative risk is 4 times higher in exposed patients than unexposed patients. While this sounds like a large amount, the attributable risk (i.e., the actual risk difference) is only 3 in 10,000 (which is 0.03%)

The statistical analysis strategy for cohort studies can be performed in *three tiers* or steps:

1. First, descriptive statistics should be used to gain an understanding of the cohort's (and the comparison cohort, when applicable) demographics as well as any baseline, clinical, and outcome variables of interest. Routine descriptive statistics for each variable can be performed as described in Chap. 1 of this text.
2. Second, bivariable statistics can be performed to evaluate for any relationships between those baseline and clinical variables. This allows the investigator to get a broad understanding of the data and inform higher-level analyses. In comparative cohort studies, this can include analysis of the exposure and outcome of interest, but also should include comparison between the cohorts for any differences in baseline demographics, clinical characteristics, length of follow-up, or other clinically meaningful covariables that may introduce bias or confounding. As outlined in Chaps. 2, 3, and 7, covariables that are associated with both the exposure and outcome of interest can confound results. An observed outcome may be due to a baseline difference between the cohorts other than the exposure of interest and, therefore, must be considered during data analysis.
3. Third, depending on the findings of step 2 and the sample size, additional regression analyses can be performed which allow the investigator to study associations between exposure and outcome while controlling for possible confounders. Broadly, logistic regression is used for binary outcomes (Chap. 2), while linear regression is used for continuous outcomes (Chap. 3). In the event that a covariable is noted to be significantly associated with both the exposure and the outcome, it must be controlled in a regression analysis as a potential confounder.

Finally, it is essential to note that cohort studies, even when prospective and comparative, are observational (not experimental) studies. Therefore, any significant associations observed must be stated as associations, and exposures should not be stated nor implied to be causative (even if an appropriate temporal relationship exists).

Analytical Review

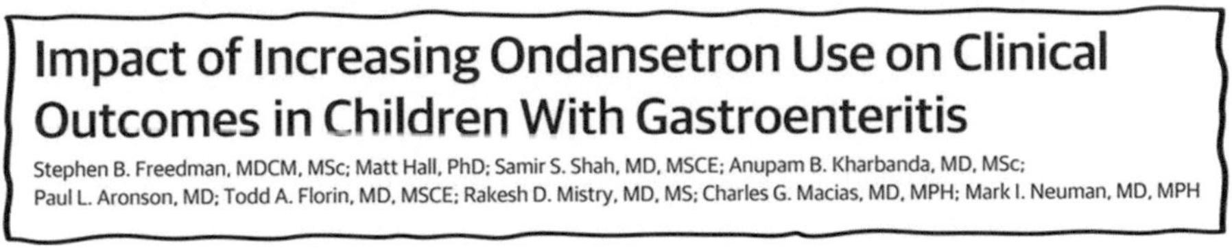

Impact of Increasing Ondansetron Use on Clinical Outcomes in Children With Gastroenteritis

Stephen B. Freedman, MDCM, MSc; Matt Hall, PhD; Samir S. Shah, MD, MSCE; Anupam B. Kharbanda, MD, MSc; Paul L. Aronson, MD; Todd A. Florin, MD, MSCE; Rakesh D. Mistry, MD, MS; Charles G. Macias, MD, MPH; Mark I. Neuman, MD, MPH

Fig. 10.3 Illustrative example of a retrospective cohort study by Freedman SB, et al. [1]

An example of a retrospective cohort study is illustrated in (Fig. 10.3).

In their 2014 study, Freedman and colleagues retrospectively investigated the effect of ondansetron use (exposure) on concomitant intravenous (IV) rehydration (outcome) for children with acute gastroenteritis [1]. The study population consisted of children under 18 years old with discharge diagnosis codes consistent with acute gastroenteritis. Their deidentified data was obtained from the Pediatric Health Information System, an administrative database that included data from 18 children's hospitals. Given the rise of ondansetron use in emergency departments in this population, this retrospective cohort study compared the rate of IV rehydration in children with acute gastroenteritis who received or did not receive ondansetron. Since the study intended to compare the outcomes of patients administered varying doses of ondansetron, a comparative cohort study was the appropriate study design.

The study population was divided into 3 cohorts: low (<5%), medium (5%–25%), and high (>25%) ondansetron use. Patients were placed in one of the 3 cohorts if the overall ondansetron use at their institution was in the specified range within a 3-month period from their encounter. Of the 804,000 patient visits analyzed, 232,706, 237,030, and 334,264 visits satisfied the low, medium, and high ondansetron uses, respectively. In their adjusted time-series analysis, the study team found no association between increasing ondansetron use and IV rehydration or hospitalization.

The authors concluded that although ondansetron use increased during the study period, IV rehydration rates were unchanged. Most children who were administered IV fluids did not receive oral ondansetron. Therefore, they identified a need to focus efforts to administer ondansetron specifically to those children at greatest risk for oral rehydration failure.

Analytical Review

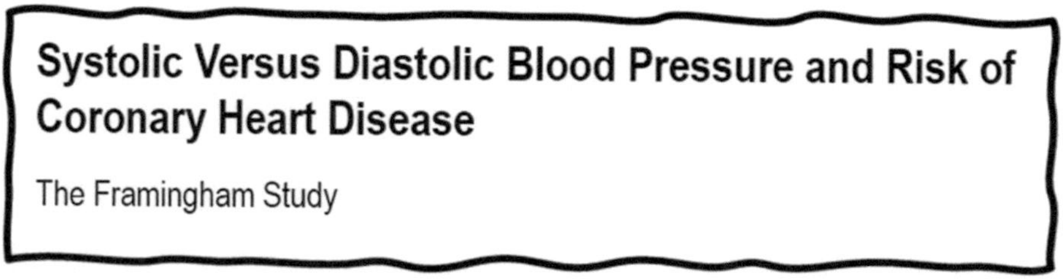

Systolic Versus Diastolic Blood Pressure and Risk of Coronary Heart Disease

The Framingham Study

Fig. 10.4 Illustrative example of a prospective cohort study by Kannel WB, et al. [2]

An example of a prospective cohort study is illustrated in (Fig. 10.4).

The Framingham study is perhaps one of the most famous and influential prospective cohort studies, which resulted in numerous changes in policy and clinical practice. In their 1971 study, Kannel and colleagues used the Framingham cohort to investigate the relationship between blood pressure (exposure) and the development of coronary heart disease (outcome) [2]. Prior to that time, the relationship between blood pressure and coronary heart disease was largely unquantified.

The study team prospectively enrolled 5,127 individuals in Framingham, MA aged 30–62 years old who did not have preexisting coronary heart disease. The participants were followed and evaluated once every two years for other known risk factors and to assess whether the participant developed clinical coronary heart disease. A prospective cohort study was the ideal study design because the research question involves the development of an outcome in individuals who were otherwise healthy at enrollment. A prospective study with a strict follow-up protocol ensures not only that participants will be enrolled independently of their eventual development coronary heart disease (limiting selection bias), but also that the collected data will be consistent and comparable among participants. Fourteen years after the cohort study began, 491 individuals in the study developed coronary heart disease.

The study team found that high blood pressure was significantly associated with coronary heart disease and suggested the importance of screening for and treating high blood pressure. Although this is considered common knowledge today, at the time of the study it was a novel finding. While it may be argued that creating the cohort from a single geographic location may have limited generalizability of the study results, it improved participant tracking, therefore, minimizing the risk of loss to follow-up. This finding led to larger multicenter studies to confirm the relationship between blood pressure and coronary heart disease.

References

1. Freedman SB, Hall M, Shah SS, et al. Impact of increasing ondansetron use on clinical outcomes in children with gastroenteritis. JAMA Pediatr. 2014;168:321–9. https://doi.org/10.1001/jamapediatrics.2013.4906.
2. Kannel WB, Gordon T, Schwartz MJ. Systolic versus diastolic blood pressure and risk of coronary heart disease. The Framingham study. Am J Cardiol. 1971;27:335–46. https://doi.org/10.1016/0002-9149(71)90428-0.

Chapter 11
Cross-Sectional Studies

Cross-sectional studies	
Pros	Cons
Quick to perform	Unable to investigate temporal or causal relationships
Inexpensive	
No additional follow-up is required	

Study Mechanics

Cross-sectional studies are observational studies in which the investigator records the exposure(s) and outcome(s) at a single time point. Unlike patients in case-control studies (Chap. 9) who are selected based on an outcome or in cohort studies (Chap. 10) who are selected based on an exposure, patients in cross-sectional studies who meet inclusion and exclusion criteria at a single point in time are identified based on any number of a variety of data points (outcome, exposure, and/or covariables).

Cross-sectional study designs are used frequently when mining epidemiologic datasets or performing surveys of a population of interest. The main advantages of cross-sectional studies are that they can be performed quickly and are inexpensive. However, exposure and outcome are collected at a single timepoint. Therefore, temporal and causal relationships may not be established. Instead, they can be preliminary investigations used to develop and refine targeted research questions for a prospective or longitudinal study. They can also be used to estimate the prevalence of exposure and disease and investigate for any associations between them.

It is important to understand how the inability to determine temporal relationships between exposure and outcome can be problematic with cross-sectional studies. Consider, for example, a cross-sectional study investigating the relationship between diet/exercise and high blood pressure. One would expect that those with

P. D. Fabricant, *Practical Clinical Research Design and Application*, https://doi.org/10.1007/978-3-031-58380-3_11

healthier diet/exercise regimens would have lower blood pressure. Because data is being collected at a single time point, the study could capture individuals with high blood pressure who have very recently started eating a healthy diet and exercising under the direction of their healthcare provider. No temporal relationship is established in a cross-sectional study; thus, it may appear as though participants with elevated blood pressure have the best diet and exercise habits. This is likely an inaccurate finding and one that might be true only for a small portion of the sample. Consequently, there may be two situations linked with high blood pressure: those study participants who have poor diet and exercise and those participants who only recently have switched to a healthy diet and exercise regimen but their blood pressure has not yet improved. This subtlety is difficult to detect and may serve to bias the result of the study toward the null (i.e., underestimate an association between exposure and outcome). Investigators must be cautious when interpreting associations (or lack of associations) when using a cross-sectional study design.

Due to data collection at a single timepoint, cross-sectional studies can measure prevalence (all currently existing cases of a disease) but not incidence (newly diagnosed cases of a disease or cases per unit time). Moreover, prevalence depends on the incidence of the disease as well as the length of survival following the outcome. If a particular condition is short-lived, either due to rapid patient recovery or death, then prevalence (at a single point in time) will be low, which may underestimate the societal burden of disease. Prevalence may be increasing or decreasing, but that will not be detected by a cross-sectional study.

Intrinsically, cross-sectional studies are most prone to selection bias. This is particularly true for queries of large administrative datasets that have already been aggregated. Because the study sample consists of all members of a population of interest who meet inclusion and exclusion criteria, selection of the appropriate population of interest is necessary to achieve a balanced representative sample. Furthermore, it is imperative that the characteristics (e.g., demographics) of the study participants included and analyzed are no different than those who were not included or refused to participate. This helps minimize concerns surrounding selection bias and an imbalanced study sample.

Special Circumstances

By definition, cross-sectional studies use data collected at a single point in time. These can include surveys, large population studies, or administrative database studies. Conversely, retrospective cohort studies involve aggregating longitudinal clinical data at a single point in time. Differences between these two study types can be confusing and are illustrated using examples below.

Consider an investigation that analyzes changes in the frequency of osteoporotic hip fractures in elderly patients over the past 20 years using a hospital admission dataset. Even though the study is describing a trend over time, each observation in the database involves a single patient whose injury is measured at a single point in time. The study design is therefore considered cross-sectional.

This is different than a retrospective analysis of prospectively collected longitudinal data. An example of this would be a chart review or secondary analysis of prospectively collected data set that was created for another research question. Although the study being performed is aggregating the data at a single point in time, because the participants were followed longitudinally during the data collection period, this should be considered a retrospective cohort study. Thus, in general, the main difference between cross-sectional studies and retrospective cohort studies is how the original data was collected.

Ideal Scenario for Cross-Sectional Study Design

The ideal scenarios for a cross-sectional design include:

- Calculating prevalence of a disease or condition in a population of interest
- Performing an initial investigation to quantify associations between exposure and outcome in order to help develop a prospective cohort study
- Answering a research question quickly and inexpensively that does not require longitudinal follow-up

Statistical Analysis

Statistical analysis for a cross-sectional study may be as simple as providing descriptive statistics on prevalence of exposure and/or disease or as complex as any other study type depending on the associations being investigated.

Like cohort studies, the statistical analysis strategy for cross-sectional studies can be performed in *three tiers* or steps:

1. First, at the most basic level, descriptive statistics can be used to report the findings of a survey, present the study sample's demographics, and determine the prevalence of any exposure(s) or outcome(s) of interest. Descriptive statistics can be reported as described in Chap. 1 and frequently answer the study question without further analyses.
2. Second, bivariable statistics can be performed to investigate for any relationships between exposure(s) and outcome(s). This can also include comparison between subgroups (e.g., those with vs. without disease) for any differences in baseline demographics or other clinical characteristics of interest. As outlined in Chapts. 2, 3, and 7, covariables that are associated with both the exposure and outcome of interest can confound results. An observed outcome may be due to a baseline difference between the cohorts other than the exposure of interest. Therefore, it must be considered during data analysis.

3. Third, depending on the findings of step 2, additional regression analyses can be performed. This allows the investigator to study associations between exposure(s) and outcome(s) while controlling for possible confounders. Broadly, logistic regression is used for binary outcomes (Chap. 2), while linear regression is used for continuous outcomes (Chap. 3). If a covariable is noted to be significantly associated with both the exposure and the outcome, it must be controlled in a regression analysis. This ensures it is not a confounding variable. However, it must be noted that the lack of a temporal relationship limits the strength of conclusions drawn from even these higher-level analyses in cross-sectional studies.

Analytical Review

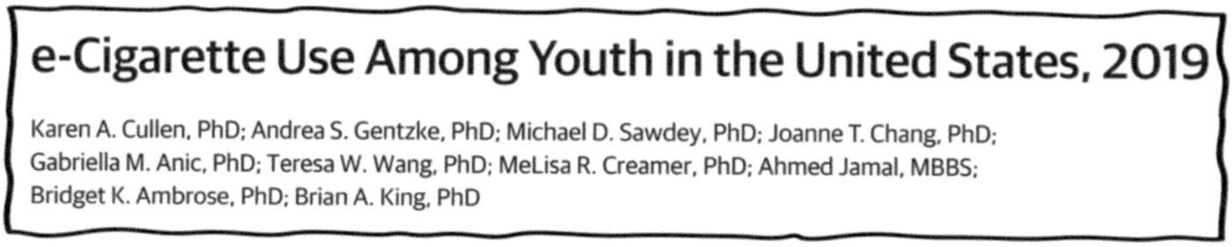

e-Cigarette Use Among Youth in the United States, 2019

Karen A. Cullen, PhD; Andrea S. Gentzke, PhD; Michael D. Sawdey, PhD; Joanne T. Chang, PhD; Gabriella M. Anic, PhD; Teresa W. Wang, PhD; MeLisa R. Creamer, PhD; Ahmed Jamal, MBBS; Bridget K. Ambrose, PhD; Brian A. King, PhD

Fig. 11.1 Illustrative example of a cross-sectional study by Cullen KA, et al. [1].

An example of a cross-sectional study is illustrated in (Fig. 11.1).

In their 2019 study, Cullen and colleagues investigated the prevalence of e-cigarette use among high school and middle school students in the United States [1]. In the years preceding this study, e-cigarette use among children had increased significantly. Given that many e-cigarette products contain high levels of nicotine, the possible effect on learning, memory, and attention is a public health concern. This study sought to quantify and describe e-cigarette use in high school and middle school students to possibly find intervention strategies to decrease consumption.

Over a four-month period, 19,018 students were asked to complete a survey that asked about frequency of e-cigarette use and brand/flavor preferences. Of the 10,019 that responded, 27.5% of high school students and 10.5% of middle school students reported e-cigarette use in the previous 30 days. Among the e-cigarette users, 34.2% of high school students and 18.0% of middle school students reported frequent use, and 59.1% of high school students and 54.1% of middle school students reported using the JUUL as the brand that they use most frequently. In addition, 72.2% of high school and 59.2% of middle school e-cigarette users smoked e-cigarettes with the following flavors: fruit (66.1%), menthol or mint (57.3%), and candy, desserts, or other sweets (34.9%).

A cross-sectional study was the appropriate design because the investigators were interested in determining the prevalence of e-cigarette use at a single point in time. When estimating the prevalence of a behavior such as e-cigarette use, it was critical for the sample to be as representative as possible. The survey used in the study by Cullen and colleagues was distributed to students chosen based on a 3-stage sampling technique intended to maintain adequate representation at the county, school, and classroom level. However, limitations inherent to cross-sectional survey studies were present: only 53% of those asked to participate filled out the survey. This may have biased the data because those who were users may have not wanted to participate. Similarly, those who replied may have denied or underreported their use, which is a common limitation of survey studies investigating known undesirable behaviors. However, both of these limitations, if anything, would have biased the results to underestimate the true prevalence of e-cigarette use in high school and middle school students. The true prevalence is therefore likely even greater than that reported in the study. The investigators' inquiry about preferred brands and flavors may serve as a starting point for policies that limit availability of certain products that are favored by underage consumers (e.g., candy or dessert flavors). Finally, after any such intervention, a similar cross-sectional survey in the same demographic may provide early evidence of its effectiveness.

Reference

1. Cullen KA, Gentzke AS, Sawdey MD, et al. E-cigarette use among youth in the United States. JAMA. 2019;322:2095–103. https://doi.org/10.1001/jama.2019.18387.

Chapter 12
Case Series and Case Reports

Case series and case reports	
Pros	Cons
Quick and inexpensive to perform	Low statistical power
Can identify a topic for further investigation	Low likelihood of changing clinical practice
	May not be generalizable

Study Mechanics

Case series (comprising five or more patients) and case reports (fewer than five patients) are the result of prospective or retrospective reporting of a single cohort of patients. Unlike comparative cohort studies, case series and case reports have few patients and a single cohort, so they do not typically include comparative statistical analyses. Rather, they report results either in narrative form or with patient-level outcomes or descriptive group statistics. They are intended to provide a unique clinical observation or experience that can heighten clinician awareness or knowledge about a unique clinical condition, innovative treatment strategy, rare complication, or an unexpected outcome.

Case series and case reports are classified as "level IV" evidence. When utilized appropriately, they are vital to the collective body of peer-reviewed literature. Specifically, they are ideal for reporting rare clinical entities, outcomes, or complications, for disseminating early clinical results from a new intervention or treatment technique, or for pilot data from which one may design and power larger prospective studies.

Retrospective case series and case reports typically begin as a series of clustered clinical observations or outcomes This sparks interest in looking back at a cohort of patients to determine the frequency of that outcome or to explore variables that may

P. D. Fabricant, *Practical Clinical Research Design and Application*, https://doi.org/10.1007/978-3-031-58380-3_12

be associated with that outcome. This typically prompts search and review of electronic health records to identify a small cohort of patients. The cohort is then reviewed, examined, and reported. The main limitation of case series and case reports is the lack of a comparison group (and therefore, comparative statistics) from which to draw conclusions about associations, risk factors, or potential causation. Despite that limitation, retrospective case series and case reports are essential for reporting rare outcomes or complications and can provide pilot data to power prospective research.

Ideal Scenario for Case Series and Case Reports

As discussed above, the ideal scenario for case series and case reports is to describe rare outcomes or complications, to disseminate early clinical results from a new intervention or treatment technique, or to procure pilot data from which one may develop larger prospective studies. It is the ideal mechanism to disseminate infrequent or clustered observations to notify other clinicians of unusual outcomes or to provide simple descriptive statistics from which a power calculation may be performed for a larger prospective comparative cohort study or randomized controlled trial.

On the contrary, case series and case reports are not appropriate for inferring causation or determining risk factors or associations with a given outcome, as there is no comparison group and the sample size is typically small. To that end, care must be taken when drawing conclusions from these studies beyond identifying topics for future research, disseminating critical and otherwise unavailable clinical information, or possibly pausing a clinical treatment with a cluster of unexpected complications.

Statistical Analysis

Statistical reporting for case series and case reports should be simple and straightforward. Frequently, for reports with few patients, patient-level data is reported in tabular format. When appropriate, each patient comprises a row with column variables that chart pertinent demographic and clinical variables and occasionally, a small narrative which describes the outcome of that patient. For larger case series, descriptive statistics may be utilized for continuous and count variables. It is important to exercise caution when reporting continuous variables. Nonparametric techniques (e.g., medians and interquartile ranges) should be used with small cohorts and non-normally distributed data because means and standard deviations may be substantially skewed by outlier data. No comparison cohort is included for analysis; therefore, comparative statistics are not appropriate in case series and case reports.

Analytical Review

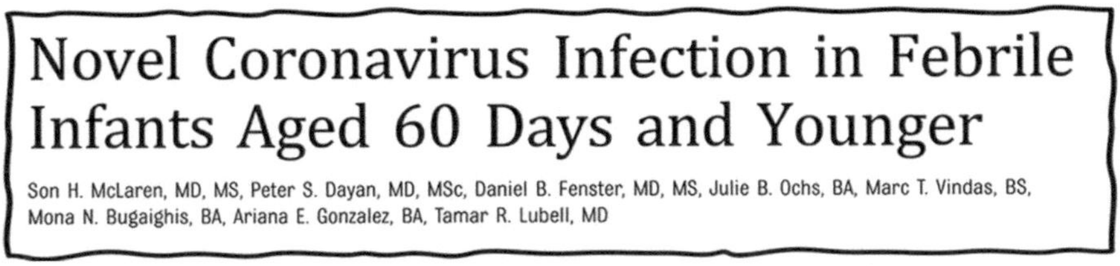

Novel Coronavirus Infection in Febrile Infants Aged 60 Days and Younger

Son H. McLaren, MD, MS, Peter S. Dayan, MD, MSc, Daniel B. Fenster, MD, MS, Julie B. Ochs, BA, Marc T. Vindas, BS, Mona N. Bugaighis, BA, Ariana E. Gonzalez, BA, Tamar R. Lubell, MD

Fig. 12.1 Illustrative example of a case series by McLaren et al. [1]

An example of an ideal use of case series methodology and reporting study is illustrated in (Fig. 12.1).

In their 2020 case series, McLaren and colleagues reported the clinical course of seven febrile infants 60 days old and younger with confirmed COVID-19 infection [1]. In March of 2020, the COVID-19 pandemic was beginning in the US, and at that time little was known about the nuances of the virus. Substantial attention and resources were being poured into treating adult patients with COVID-19 infection; however, the clinical presentation and outcomes in infants were unknown. At their large urban academic children's hospital in New York City where there were early outbreaks, the authors were in a unique position to gather initial data on COVID-19 infection in young infants who were at high risk of developing respiratory complications or invasive bacterial infections in the setting of fever.

In the first 6 weeks of the pandemic, the authors compiled data on seven febrile patients aged 60 days and younger who tested positive for SARS-CoV-2, a virus which causes COVID-19. They noted that unlike adults, young infants with COVID-19 often had mild illness, similar to typical viral illness with other coronaviruses in this demographic. The rapid dissemination of this data is evident in the published study timeline. Data was collected from March 1 to April 15, 2020. Then the publication was drafted, submitted, and accepted on June 1, 2020. Approximately 3 months after the first infant presented to the hospital, the manuscript was available online on June 11, 2020.

In the early days of the COVID-19 pandemic, any helpful clinical information was vital to broadcast quickly. A case series is the most appropriate study design in such a scenario. A long-term prospective study would be too time consuming, and any experimental study design would be impossible. Results from this study, which were supported by other case series, provided timely data to help clinicians make more informed decisions. Certainly, longer-term follow-up and more rigorous investigation using a larger study sample were imperative throughout the pandemic and continued for many studies which were initiated during this period.

Analytical Review

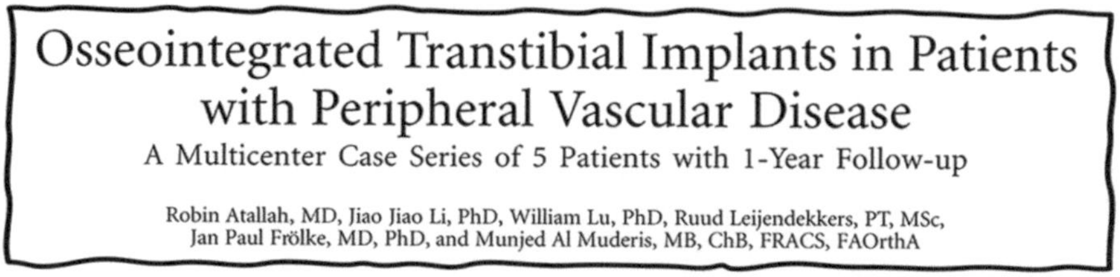

Osseointegrated Transtibial Implants in Patients with Peripheral Vascular Disease

A Multicenter Case Series of 5 Patients with 1-Year Follow-up

Robin Atallah, MD, Jiao Jiao Li, PhD, William Lu, PhD, Ruud Leijendekkers, PT, MSc,
Jan Paul Frölke, MD, PhD, and Munjed Al Muderis, MB, ChB, FRACS, FAOrthA

Fig. 12.2 Illustrative example of a case series by Atallah et al. [2]

An example of an ideal use of case series methodology and reporting study is illustrated in (Fig. 12.2).

In their 2017 case series, Atallah and colleagues utilized a case series to report the one-year outcomes of five patients who underwent an osseointegration procedure for limb reconstruction after transtibial amputation [2]. At the time, osseointegration was considered an alternative treatment for amputees who were not able to wear a standard socket prosthesis. In an osseointegration procedure, instead of a socket prosthesis coupling externally to the limb stump, a device is implanted directly into the bone and extends through the skin and outside the body. Then, prosthetic lower limb segments can be attached to the external portion of the osseointegration prosthesis. Although peripheral vascular disease is the cause of most lower limb amputations, at the time of publication, peripheral vascular disease was considered a relative contraindication for osseointegration, which had mainly been used to reconstruct traumatic limb loss.

Since there was limited data to support the use of osseointegration in patients with peripheral vascular disease and the procedure in this population was rarely performed, the investigators pooled together five patients from their respective institutions to describe the one-year outcomes after osseointegration. They noted that the mobility of all five patients improved, and four of the five patients were pain-free at 1 year after surgery. Despite three of the five patients being wheelchair-bound before the procedure, all five patients were able to walk and perform activities of daily living at follow-up. There were two cases of superficial soft tissue infections, but no deep infections, implant loosening, or implant failures.

The authors appropriately reported each of the five patients' demographic, preoperative clinical information, and outcomes in tabular format without drawing any comparisons or forming any causative arguments. Rather, the authors concluded that "osseointegrated implants can be an effective treatment for transtibial amputees with peripheral vascular disease and can result in benefits, including improved function and mobility." They further advised that "additional evidence is required to confirm the feasibility of implementing osseointegration surgery as standard care for amputees with peripheral vascular disease" and that "larger prospective studies with longer follow-up are necessary to accurately examine the effects of osseointegration surgery in this patient cohort."

This early case series correctly avoided drawing overreaching conclusions beyond what their data demonstrated. Instead, they identified a patient demographic that could benefit from this historically overlooked procedure, illustrated the limitations of their investigation, and suggested an area of future prospective comparative research to further evaluate this treatment option in patients with peripheral vascular disease.

References

1. McLaren SH, Dayan PS, Fenster DB, et al. Novel coronavirus infection in febrile infants aged 60 days and younger. Pediatrics. 2020;146:e20201550. https://doi.org/10.1542/peds.2020-1550.
2. Atallah R, Li JJ, Lu W, et al. Osseointegrated transtibial implants in patients with peripheral vascular disease: a multicenter case series of 5 patients with 1-year follow-up. J Bone Joint Surg Am. 2017;99:1516–23. https://doi.org/10.2106/JBJS.16.01295.

Part III
Specialized Study Designs

Chapter 13
Propensity Score-Matched Studies

Propensity score-matched studies	
Pros	Cons
Exchangeability is achieved without randomization	Only controls for measured covariables
Use of a single propensity score (instead of multiple covariables) allows for the inclusion of many covariables without the restrictions of multivariable modeling	Requires large samples to balance the covariables
Sample may be more representative of real-world patients rather than those who would have been randomized	Group overlap is needed to have sufficient patients to create exchangeable groups
	Any missing data gives a missing propensity score; therefore, patients with any missing data must be excluded

Study Mechanics

In clinical research, the optimal study investigating an exposure–outcome relationship is one that compares two groups that are as similar as possible on all variables except the exposure of interest. If the two groups have identical characteristics except the exposure of interest, then they are referred to as "exchangeable." Exchangeability is the measurement of comparability between treatment groups and is essential to causal inference between exposure and outcome. In randomized controlled trials (RCTs) (Chap. 8), the probability of exposure (or treatment intervention) in a two-group study is 0.5. In that scenario, with large enough groups, there is maximal exchangeability. Each group is the same on all variables except for the exposure or treatment assignment. This includes variables that may be considered potential confounders (e.g., age, sex, and body mass index) as well as any that are seemingly irrelevant (e.g., eye color). Furthermore, randomization of a large

© The Author(s), under exclusive license to Springer Nature Switzerland AG 2024

P. D. Fabricant, *Practical Clinical Research Design and Application*, https://doi.org/10.1007/978-3-031-58380-3_13

group of study participants creates balanced groups of variables that are unknown and, perhaps, not even measurable. This protects the findings of an RCT against future research by balancing potential confounders of the exposure–outcome relationship that were not considered initially. With a large enough study cohort, any quantifiable or nonquantifiable variable should be balanced between exposure and treatment groups. This creates exchangeability.

However, in observational studies, the probability of group assignment is not random. Patients may be assigned treatment (i.e., exposure) based on clinical decisions that take certain patient characteristics into account. This introduces confounding and limits exchangeability between study groups. There are also instances in which an experimental study is not feasible or ethical. Propensity score matching (PSM) was described by Rosenbaum and Rubin to create more exchangeable cohorts for comparison [1]. This method, rather than regression analysis (Chaps. 2 and 3), can control confounders and can also estimate a potential causal effect of exposure on an outcome when using observational data. However, residual confounding is possible for any unmeasured variable not included in the PSM methodology. Furthermore, PSM cannot make up for missing data or poor data accuracy. This is sometimes problematic with observational or retrospective studies but is not problematic in a prospective experimental design. Therefore, the statistical rigor of studies using PSM falls between observational and experimental study designs.

When performing a study using PSM, the investigator must first decide on the list of covariables with which to perform propensity matching. Ideally, these variables are a comprehensive list of predictors associated with treatment (exposure) but not related to the outcome. Then, the investigator uses logistic regression to calculate a propensity score for each patient. The "propensity" describes the likelihood that a patient received the treatment, given the values of the covariables in aggregate. Next, patients from each treatment group are matched based on their propensity score, rather than on the individual variables that underlie it. This way, the propensity score balances the identified covariables on the whole, and the distribution of observed baseline covariables should be similar between treated and untreated (or alternatively-treated) patients. Matching of patients is done by pairing patients from each treatment group with the closest propensity scores within certain caliper bounds (which is a limit of how far apart they can be). Patients without a match are discarded from analysis. Minimizing the number of patients excluded for this reason is important to avoid introducing bias into the cohort. The number of matches can be maximized by widening the caliper ranges. However, if they are too wide (e.g., matches that are farther apart are considered acceptable), the resulting cohorts may not be exchangeable. Typically, 1% (0.01) is chosen as a cutoff to optimize the exchangeability between groups and include as many matches as possible.

After PSM has been performed, it is important to check the balance of the underlying covariables between groups. Ideally, there should be less than a 10% difference of the individual covariables between treatment (exposure) groups. Larger differences may indicate that the groups are not exchangeable. Statistical analysis may proceed once the investigator confirms acceptable exchangeability of the treatment groups.

Ideal Scenario for Propensity Score-Matched Studies

The ideal scenario for a PSM design is one with a large dataset from which to construct balanced cohorts. There should be a strong overlap of covariables (and therefore propensity scores). Patients with outlier propensity scores cannot be included in the study, and there is an increasing risk of bias with an increasing number of patients who are not included. Ideal data sources include multicenter registries and prospective study datasets which can be analyzed secondarily using PSM methodology. However, PSM methodology cannot overcome data quality concerns; therefore, data sources must be thoroughly scrutinized.

Statistical Analysis

Since PSM methodology creates pairs of patients (one from each treatment group), paired analyses are typically most appropriate. Practically, this can be thought of as a mean of differences in outcomes between treatment group pairs. These are covered elsewhere (Chaps. 2 and 3) and include analyses such as the McNemar test (a paired chi-squared test) and paired samples t-tests. Higher-level paired regression analyses include conditional logistic regression analysis and are beyond the scope of this text.

Conclusion

In conclusion, PSM helps to reduce selection bias and improves the comparability of treatment groups in observational studies by creating exchangeable treatment groups. Unlike randomized controlled studies, it does not equally distribute additional unknown, unobserved variables between treatment groups. The investigator should carefully consider potential unobserved confounders because the validity of the results depends on the exchangeability between treatment groups. The more similar the treatment groups (except on the treatment or exposure), the more valid the results of the study.

Analytical Review

Weight recurrence after Sleeve Gastrectomy versus Roux-en-Y gastric bypass: a propensity score matched nationwide analysis

Erman O. Akpinar · Ronald S. L. Liem · Simon W. Nienhuijs · Jan Willem M. Greve ·
Perla J. Marang-van de Mheen · on behalf of the Dutch Audit for Treatment of Obesity Research Group

Fig. 13.1 Illustrative example of a propensity score-matched study by Akpinar et al. [2]

An example of a propensity score-matched study is illustrated in (Fig. 13.1).

In 2022, Akpinar and colleagues conducted a study utilizing PSM to investigate the extent of weight gain recurrence between patients who underwent sleeve gastrectomy (SG) versus Roux-en-Y gastric bypass (RYGB). Previous studies had compared weight recurrence in these two groups but had not appropriately adjusted for confounders.

To perform their study, the investigators included patients undergoing either SG or RYGB between 2015 and 2018 using data from the Dutch Audit for Treatment of Obesity (DATO). Prior to matching, there were differences in important baseline characteristics such as age, sex, body mass index, American Society of Anesthesiologists Classification, prevalence of type II diabetes, hypertension, dyslipidemia, gastroesophageal reflux disease, obstructive sleep apnea, and osteoarthritis. Given the underlying differences between treatment groups, any of these covariables could confound an observed relationship between treatment and weight gain recurrence. After PSM was performed, no differences in these baseline characteristics were present in the cohort for analysis. Furthermore, before matching, there were 4,780 SG patients and 14,982 RYGB patients. After matching, there were 4,693 in each group. This resulted in balanced, exchangeable groups with 1:1 matching and included 98.2% of the overall SG cohort.

With these exchangeable groups, the investigators discovered that patients who underwent SG were more likely to experience weight gain recurrence between 2 and 5 years following surgery. Also, they were less likely to achieve comorbidity remission than those who underwent RYGB. The authors concluded that when considered in the context of a shared decision-making process (to include additional factors such as risk of complications or revision surgery), RYGB is preferred over SG based on lower frequency of weight gain recurrence and more frequent comorbidity remission.

This study showcases the proper implementation of PSM methodology. First, the investigators identified a large, high-quality dataset and calculated propensity scores. Second, they matched patients 1:1 based on the propensity scores and utilized almost all of the patients in the smaller treatment group. Third, they confirmed the balance of potential confounders and quality of the propensity score match prior to appropriately analyzing the propensity-matched cohort.

References

1. Rosenbaum PR, Rubin DB. The central role of the propensity score in observational studies for causal effects. Biometrika. 1983;70:41–55. https://doi.org/10.1093/biomet/70.1.41.
2. Akpinar EO, Liem RS, Nienhuijs SW, et al. Weight recurrence after sleeve gastrectomy versus Roux-en-Y gastric bypass: a propensity score matched nationwide analysis. Surg Endosc. 2023;37:4351–9. https://doi.org/10.1007/s00464-022-09785-8.

Chapter 14
Interrater and Intrarater Reliability Studies

Study Mechanics

Intrarater reliability is the degree of consistency and stability of measurements made by the same rater or observer on multiple occasions when evaluating the same patients or items. Interrater reliability assesses the agreement or consistency between two or more different raters or observers when they independently assess or measure the same patients or items. Both are essential to ensure the dependability and consistency of observational data, and quantifying these metrics requires a formal reliability study.

To perform an interrater and intrarater reliability study, an investigator identifies cases to be evaluated, selects one or more measurements to be calculated, and enrolls multiple raters to perform the measurements. There is no universally accepted number of cases or raters needed to perform a reliability study; however, at least 50 cases are typically evaluated by three or more raters. If reliability scores are suboptimal, by including multiple raters an investigator can probe into why that might be the case. For instance, there might be one rater whose scores are outliers compared to the rest of the raters, or there may be widespread variability in ratings among all the raters. How each of these scenarios is addressed varies based on the underlying cause of low reliability.

For example, let's consider a newly described magnetic resonance imaging (MRI) scoring system for knee arthritis. Such a scoring system may look at several elements when assessing the knee: cartilage, the underlying bone, additional soft tissue structures, and the overall health of the joint. This system may output a continuous, ordinal, or binary score for cartilage health.

First, the investigator should identify 50 or more knee MRIs in patients across the entire spectrum of cartilage health. Then, the investigator enrolls raters with a variety of clinical backgrounds who would utilize such a score clinically. In this example, that might include radiologists, orthopedic surgeons, rheumatologists, and

P. D. Fabricant, *Practical Clinical Research Design and Application*,
https://doi.org/10.1007/978-3-031-58380-3_14

primary care doctors. It may be beneficial to enroll individuals at varying levels of training (e.g., students, residents, fellows, and attendings).

The investigator then teaches the MRI scoring system to the raters. Once all raters have been instructed on the scoring system, they begin rating the knee MRIs. All raters proceed scoring all of the MRIs individually and submit their scores to the investigator. Then, at a later date, the same raters score the same MRIs. This is done in random order and at a duration long enough after the first round of rating (typically 2 weeks or longer) to minimize the risk of score recall (Fig. 14.1).

The investigator then proceeds with statistical analysis (discussed in the next section). If both interrater and intrarater reliability are acceptable, then the score is considered reliable. Additional validity testing might be performed (discussed in Chap. 15) to determine if the score is clinically predictive of disease (which, in this example, is knee arthritis).

If the interrater reliability is suboptimal, the investigator should do a deeper dive to evaluate for potential causes. If a single rater or small subgroup of raters had outlier scores, then they can be retrained prior to rescoring the MRIs. If individuals with certain expertise or subspecialty training demonstrated outlier scores, it may be that specialized training or additional expertise is required to appropriately use the score. If the scores were inconsistent (with many outliers due to unpredictable reasons), the scoring system may require changes in its design.

Similarly, if the intrarater reliability is suboptimal, the investigator should evaluate for an underlying reason. If reliability was low for a single rater or small subset of raters, the investigator should inquire into any different conditions at the time of the second rating that may have affected the scores (e.g., equipment, mood, fatigue). Importantly, acceptable intrarater reliability is one required component of achieving satisfactory interrater reliability, since consistency of each rater over time is generally required to have consistency among a group of raters for a measurement designed to be used frequently.

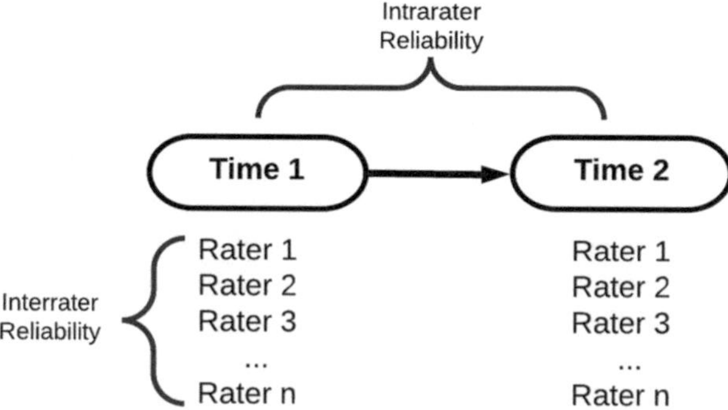

Fig. 14.1 To conduct an interrater and intrarater reliability study, ratings are performed on all cases by each rater at two distinct time points. Interrater reliability is the measurement of agreement among the raters, while intrarater reliability is the agreement of measurements made by the same rater when evaluating the same items at different times

Statistical Analysis

Statistical analysis for reliability testing is performed based on the structure of the data (e.g., continuous, ordinal, binary) and the number of raters. While an exhaustive list of reliability statistics and exact formulas are beyond the scope of this text, the most commonly used reliability tests are listed below with brief descriptions and interpretations of each test.

Percent Agreement

Percent agreement is a simple calculation of the percentage of ratings that agree. While it is easily calculated and directly interpretable, it has several limitations. First, for non-binary ratings, it cannot determine the degree of disagreement between the ratings. For example, if each rater is categorizing a variable as small, medium, or large, percent agreement does not discriminate between a disagreement between small and medium (off by one size) or small and large (off by 2 sizes). Both would be similarly scored as a disagreement.

Second, unlike kappa (discussed below), percent agreement does not take expected agreement into account. Therefore, it cannot account for guessing or the possibility of some amount of agreement occurring by chance.

Kappa

Kappa is the statistic that is used to measure interrater reliability for categorical items, including binary, ordinal, or nominal categories. Unlike percent agreement, it accounts for raters' guessing and agreement due to random chance. For this reason, it is considered to be a more robust reliability measure. Kappa values can range from 0 (agreement that is no better than chance) to 1 (perfect agreement). Negative kappa values are present when agreement is worse than chance and indicate systematic disagreement among raters.

The two most common forms of kappa are as follows:

- Cohen's kappa: The agreement between two raters who each classify N items into C mutually exclusive categories
- Fleiss' kappa: The agreement between M (greater than two) raters who each classify N items into C mutually exclusive categories

Finally, kappa may also be weighted or unweighted. Weighted kappa allows disagreements to be weighted differently. This can be thought of like getting "partial credit" for disagreements that are close. Conversely, unweighted kappa treats all disagreements the same. Therefore, weighted kappa is appropriate for ordinal scales, while unweighted kappa is appropriate for binary or nominal scales [1, 2].

Intraclass Correlation Coefficient

The intraclass correlation coefficient (ICC) quantifies the correlation within a class of data (e.g., repeated measures by different raters) and has a value between 0 and 1. There are several different versions of the ICC that can be applied depending on the clinical or experimental situation. Selecting the correct version is imperative to obtaining valid results. Although the classification described by Shrout and Fleiss predates that by McGraw and Wong, the descriptive classification by McGraw and Wong is more comprehensible and frequently used in statistical software packages, so it will be presented first [3, 4].

McGraw and Wong defined 10 forms of ICC. These variations take the experimental structure into account based on the model (one-way random effects, two-way random effects, or two-way fixed effects), the type (single rater or the mean of k raters), and whether it is important to have absolute agreement or consistency [4].

Selecting the correct ICC form can be done by answering the following four questions:

1. Will all patients be rated by the same set of raters?
2. Will the study be used to generalize the findings so that any individual with similar clinical training can use the scoring instrument (e.g., a clinical prediction rule), or will the single set of specific raters for the study be the only ones to ever use the instrument (e.g., to be used for the study only)?
3. In the clinical setting, will single ratings be used or will the mean value of multiple raters be used?
4. Is absolute agreement between raters important or is consistency of ratings (even if they do not agree) sufficient?

Model selection. The three models are as follows:

1. *One-way random effects*: In a one-way random effects model, each participant is measured by a different set of randomly selected raters. In other words, the same raters do not rate the same participants. One example of when this model would be used is during a multicenter study in which raters evaluate only the subcohort of participants from their respective centers.
2. *Two-way random effects*: In a two-way random effects model, each participant is measured by the same set of raters. These raters come from a larger population of potential raters. This model is the most commonly used for interrater reliability studies, as it is appropriate for situations in which the investigators plan to generalize their findings to other clinicians and researchers who have similar training. For instance, consider a scenario where investigators are testing a novel radiographic measurement. This measurement, performed by three radiologists participating in the reliability study, aims to be implemented for routine clinical use by all radiologists.

3. *Two-way mixed effects*: In a two-way mixed effects model, each participant is measured by a fixed number of raters. Unlike a two-way random effects model, the results cannot be generalized to other raters and represent only the reliability of the specific raters in the study. It is not commonly used because most interrater reliability studies are performed to demonstrate the reliability of a measurement or scale for use in a broader clinical or research setting.

Type selection. Two types based on number of measurements:

1. *Single measures*: In single measures, even though multiple ratings are done for the interrater reliability study, reliability is applied to the clinical context in which a single measure of a single rater will be performed and used clinically.
2. *Average measures*: In average measures, reliability is applied to the clinical context where the measures of multiple raters will be averaged for each patient.

Definition selection. Absolute agreement versus consistency:

1. *Absolute agreement*: In an absolute agreement definition, the exact agreement between raters is important (i.e., how closely the measurements agree with each other). This includes systematic errors as well as random residual errors.
2. *Consistency*: In a consistency definition, any systematic errors are discounted and the ICC calculation will only account for random residual error. In this scenario, the correlation or trend of raters is sufficient for reliability (i.e., how the raters rank or score the items relative to each other, without necessarily requiring the absolute values to be in agreement), which in the clinical setting is generally less important than absolute agreement.

With an understanding of the above concepts, one can define the six Shrout and Fleiss forms of ICC based on varying combinations of the McGraw and Wong forms [3]. The Shrout and Fleiss ICC forms (Table 14.1) are important to understand because this notation is frequently used in medical literature.

The most commonly used form of ICC for interrater reliability studies is two-way random effects with single measures and absolute agreement [ICC(2,1)]. In this form, a group of raters scores all participants with a priority on absolute agreement and the goal of demonstrating sufficient reliability. This way, the instrument can be used clinically by individuals with similar training. Notably, even though the reliability testing experiment involves multiple raters, if the instrument is designed to be used clinically by a single rater, then ICC(2,1) is selected.

Table 14.1 Shrout and Fleiss ICC forms and the corresponding McGraw and Wong model, type, and definition

Shrout and Fleiss ICC form	Model, type, and definition (McGraw and Wong)
ICC(1,1)	One-way random, single measures, absolute agreement
ICC(2,1)	Two-way random, single measures, absolute agreement
ICC(3,1)	Two-way mixed, single measures, consistency
ICC(1,k)	One-way random, average measures, absolute agreement
ICC(2,k)	Two-way random, average measures, absolute agreement
ICC(3,k)	Two-way mixed, average measures, consistency

Interpretation of Kappa and Intraclass Correlation Coefficient Values

As discussed above, kappa and ICC values range between 0 (agreement that is no better than chance) and 1 (perfect agreement). Negative kappa values are present when agreement is worse than chance and indicate systematic disagreement among raters. While they are reported numerically, it is important to know commonly accepted descriptive classifications for these values.

Perhaps the earliest and most well-known criteria for interpreting kappa values were set forth in 1977 by Landis and Koch [5]. They suggested that values from 0.00 to 0.20 indicate slight agreement, 0.21 to 0.40 indicate fair agreement, 0.41 to 0.60 indicate moderate agreement, 0.61 to 0.80 indicate substantial agreement, and 0.81 to 1.00 indicate almost perfect or perfect agreement. More recently, Cicchetti advocated expanding these criteria to ICC as well [6]. He defined them as: 0.00 to 0.39 being poor agreement, 0.40 to 0.59 being fair agreement, 0.60 to 0.74 being good agreement, and 0.75 to 1.00 being excellent agreement.

Analytical Review

> **VARIABILITY IN RADIOLOGISTS' INTERPRETATIONS OF MAMMOGRAMS**
>
> Joann G. Elmore, M.D., M.P.H., Carolyn K. Wells, M.P.H., Carol H. Lee, M.D., Debra H. Howard, M.D., and Alvan R. Feinstein, M.D.

Fig. 14.2 Illustrative example of an interrater and intrarater reliability study by Elmore et al. [7]

An example of a interrater and intrarater reliability study is illustrated in (Fig. 14.2).

In their 1994 study, Elmore and colleagues investigated the diagnostic accuracy and reliability of radiologists' interpretations of mammograms. Ten radiologists independently reviewed 150 mammograms: 27 from women with confirmed breast cancer and 123 without breast cancer. The radiologists were instructed to complete a checklist where they noted abnormalities such as a mass or calcification, the location of the abnormality, and the relative severity of the abnormality in the cases of multiple identified abnormalities. To test interrater reliability, the radiologists provided diagnoses under the following four categories: normal, abnormal but probably benign, abnormal and indeterminant, or abnormal and suggestive of cancer. Additionally, management recommendations were selected from the following list: routine mammographic follow-up, mammographic follow-up after a short interval, additional mammographic views, ultrasound examination, or biopsy. To test intrarater reliability, the radiologists performed readings in random order at two separate time points (5 months apart).

Diagnostic accuracy was determined by comparing the raters' diagnoses to patients' confirmed cancer diagnoses. Interrater reliability was assessed using weighted kappa to account for a 4-level ordinal diagnosis classification. This allowed quantification of any degree of clinical disagreement from minimal to substantial. Intrarater reliability was assessed on a subset of 50 images presented with each patient's age but no other clinical information. Although the investigators found high intrarater reliability for recommending biopsy (kappa = 0.71), interrater reliability with respect to diagnosis and suggested management was low (weighted kappa = 0.47). Finally, although some of the radiologists recommended immediate biopsy for a high percentage of patients with confirmed cancer (up to 96%), radiologists with the highest rates of immediate biopsy recommendations did so regardless of whether patients had cancer or not.

The study concluded that although mammography is of value in screening women for breast cancer, efforts to improve accuracy and reduce variability in diagnostic interpretation were needed to increase the effectiveness of mammograms for detecting early breast cancer. As discussed in Chap. 5, adequate reliability (i.e., reduced variability, increased precision) is a prerequisite for accuracy. If a test lacks precision, it has an unpredictable output. Therefore, it cannot be clinically useful (Fig. 5.2). This landmark study led to advances in imaging technology and interpretation techniques that improved the utility of mammography for detecting early-stage breast cancer.

References

1. Lantz CA. Application and evaluation of the kappa statistic in the design and interpretation of chiropractic clinical research. J Manip Physiol Ther. 1997;20:521–8.
2. Sim J, Wright CC. The kappa statistic in reliability studies: use, interpretation, and sample size requirements. Phys Ther. 2005;85:257–68. https://doi.org/10.1093/ptj/85.3.257.
3. Shrout PE, Fleiss JL. Intraclass correlations: uses in assessing rater reliability. Psychol Bull. 1979;86:420–8. https://doi.org/10.1037/0033-2909.86.2.420.
4. McGraw KO, Wong SP. Forming inferences about some intraclass correlation coefficients. Psychol Methods. 1996;1:30–46. https://doi.org/10.1037/1082-989X.1.1.30.
5. Landis JR, Koch GG. The measurement of observer agreement for categorical data. Biometrics. 1977;33:159–74. https://doi.org/10.2307/2529310.
6. Cicchetti DV. Guidelines, criteria, and rules of thumb for evaluating normed and standardized assessment instruments in psychology. Psychol Assess. 1994;6:284–90. https://doi.org/10.1037/1040-3590.6.4.284.
7. Elmore JG, Wells CK, Lee CH, et al. Variability in radiologists' interpretations of mammograms. N Engl J Med. 1994;331:1493–9. https://doi.org/10.1056/NEJM199412013312206.

Chapter 15
Clinical Outcome Scale Development and Validation

What Is a Clinical Outcome Scale?

A clinical outcome scale is an instrument that is used to assess and quantify specific aspects of a patient's health, pain, function, or symptoms. Unlike objective performance indicators, clinical outcome scales are questionnaires that are completed either by the patient, clinician, or an independent observer. Patient-reported outcome measures (PROMs) are the most commonly used clinical outcome scales and will be the focus of this chapter.

PROM questionnaires have become vital for patient care and clinical research as they provide valuable insight into the patient's own experience. They allow healthcare professionals to evaluate treatment efficacy, monitor intervention response and disease progression, compare different treatment strategies, and compare health status between patients. They can be used in clinical research studies to directly compare interventions or therapies by quantifying various patient-centered domains including pain, physical function, stress, mental health, social well-being, and satisfaction. These scales can be generic (e.g., quality of life scales such as the 36-Item Short Form Survey [SF-36], pain scales such as the Wong-Baker Faces Pain Rating Scale) or condition-specific (e.g., Oxford Knee Score, Asthma Quality of Life Questionnaire).

Patient-Reported Outcome Scale Development vs. Cross-Validation of an Existing Scale

Importantly, PROMs must be validated in the population in which they are to be used. For condition-specific PROMs, this also includes the specific condition being investigated. For example, a knee arthritis scale designed for adults should not be

P. D. Fabricant, *Practical Clinical Research Design and Application*, https://doi.org/10.1007/978-3-031-58380-3_15

applied to children or used for non-arthritic knee conditions. To that end, if no such PROM exists for the condition and population of interest, one must either be created de novo or an existing scale can be adapted through the process of cross-validation. In either case, as discussed later in this chapter, reliability and validity must be tested in the population of interest prior to using the scale clinically or for research. Reliability is a measure of the stability and consistency of the scale over time in the absence of any clinical change. Validity is the ability of a PROM to measure what it intends to measure and be unaffected by other confounding factors.

Scale Development and Pilot Testing

A formal research database search should be performed to identify if condition and population-specific PROMs exist. If the research team finds a scale that may be appropriate to use, but it has not been validated in that specific demographic or clinical condition, they may attempt to cross-validate the existing scale. In that case, they would skip the process of scale development and move on to reliability and validity testing.

Conversely, if a scale is to be developed de novo, the investigator must go through a series of initial steps to create a PROM that will be assessed for reliability and validity. This process involves the following steps:

1. *Item Generation:* The process of item generation serves to identify a comprehensive list of items to be considered for inclusion in the PROM. A group of stakeholders are surveyed to generate a list of items to be considered for inclusion in the PROM. These stakeholders can be patients, physicians, nurses, physical therapists, and others. In addition to independently generating a list of items, any similar scales identified during the literature search are also reviewed for relevant items to consider. Surveying continues until no new responses are generated. The investigator then eliminates duplicate answers and compiles a provisional item list.

2. *Item Reduction:* During item reduction, a cohort of individuals in the target demographic is asked to score the importance of each item (e.g., on a 10-point scale) as well as the frequency with which they experience, perform, or are interested in performing that item. Summed importance and frequency scores for each item are then averaged and ranked to identify those items with the greatest relevance to the population of interest. The original clinicians involved in item generation can then re-evaluate this list for clinical sensibility to ensure the final list of items reflect the interests and priorities of both patients and clinicians.

3. *Scale Creation and Formatting:* The investigators then create the scale to incorporate those items identified to be most clinically relevant. This includes designing the layout, formulating the item wording, and creating a scoring algorithm. They should use simple and straightforward language at or below an eighth grade reading level, which can be calculated in most word processing applica-

tions using the Flesch-Kincaid grade level analysis. For pediatric patients, a lower grade reading level may be more appropriate. If needed, this allows the parent/guardian to read the item prompts so that they are comprehensible to the child.

4. *Pilot Testing:* Pilot testing is an iterative process of administering the scale to test participants in the population of interest and then soliciting feedback on item understanding, language, layout, and ease of completion. By using open-ended questions, the investigators can gain valuable insights on how to make edits to the PROM. This is done repeatedly (usually in several rounds of 5–10 participants at a time) until no additional feedback is provided.

After this process is complete, the investigators have a novel PROM on which to perform reliability and validity testing.

Structure of Reliability and Validity Testing

Once the scale is ready for reliability and validity testing, the study is uniquely structured as demonstrated in Fig. 15.1. In traditional hypothesis-based investigations, there is a primary hypothesis and not more than a few secondary hypotheses, if any. In outcome scale development, after ensuring reliability, the process of validation testing requires examining a list of a priori hypotheses for relationships that the investigator would expect to see are present (convergent validity) or are absent (discriminant validity). Only after all hypotheses are tested can the investigator assess the validity of the outcome scale being examined.

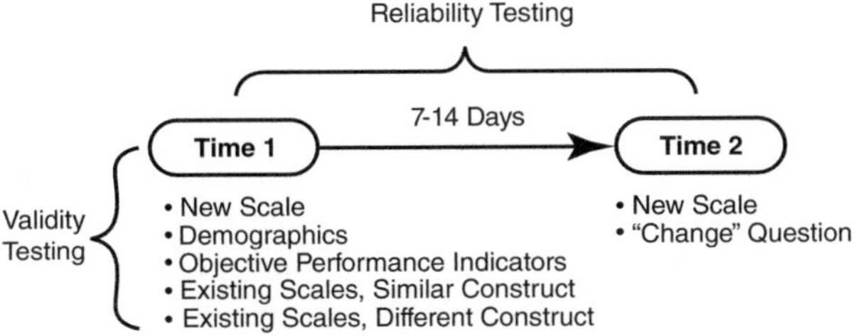

Fig. 15.1 After developing a new outcome scale (or identifying an existing scale for cross-validation), reliability and validity testing may be performed. This involves administering the new scale to a group of patients or research participants along with existing scales of similar construct (for convergent validity testing) and scales with different constructs (for discriminant validity testing). Relevant objective performance indicators are collected whenever possible to use in convergent validity testing, and baseline demographics are also frequently collected to ensure that these do not affect scale scores during discriminant validity testing. After a period of time long enough for participants to forget their responses but short enough so that their clinical condition does not change (typically 7 to14 days, but can vary based on clinical condition), patients take the new scale again and answer a "change" question. The "change" question is a single item asking the participant if anything has changed with respect to their health or clinical condition in the interim. Only those without changes in their clinical condition are included in the reliability analysis

Reliability Testing

Reliability testing includes two types of analyses:

1. *Internal consistency:* Internal consistency testing evaluates the association among multiple items in an outcome scale which are designed to measure the same construct and therefore should have a high amount of shared variance (covariance). This is most commonly calculated using Cronbach's alpha. It may also be calculated using the split-half method whereby the items are randomly split in half and the answers to each half are compared for consistency.

2. *Test–retest reliability:* Test–retest reliability examines the stability and reproducibility of the scale results over time in the absence of relevant clinical change. This is performed by administering the scale at two separate time points far enough apart to minimize the risk of answer recall, but close enough together that the patient's clinical condition has not changed. Then the scores are compared using correlation analysis or intraclass correlation coefficient (ICC). Typically, ICC with absolute agreement is preferred. It is the strictest test for reliability (discussed in Chap. 14) as it accounts for a troublesome scenario where scores can be highly correlated but do not completely agree. Take, for instance, three raters who completed a 10-point PROM under development and at time one their scores were 3, 4, and 5. Then at time two, the same raters scored 7, 8, and 9, respectively. These outcomes are highly correlated, but do not agree since each raters' score increased by 4 points between the first and second administration. ICC with absolute agreement prevents this problem by calculating on the scores' absolute agreement rather than correlation alone.

Construct Validity Testing

Construct validity is a concept that includes convergent validity and discriminant validity. Convergent validity is demonstrated when a scale is associated with similar constructs or objective performance indicators to which it would be expected to be related. Discriminant validity is demonstrated when a scale is *not* associated with *dissimilar* constructs to which it should not be related, such as baseline demographics (Fig. 15.1). Statistical testing of these hypotheses is performed using standard statistical methodology (Chaps. 2 and 3) such as *t*-tests and correlation analyses to demonstrate the presence or absence of associations for convergent and discriminant validity, respectively. For convergent validity testing using correlation analyses, moderately positive correlation values between 0.3 and 0.6 are optimal. This range indicates the presence of a statistically significant positive correlation, but one that is not so high or tightly correlated that the new scale is redundantly measuring the exact same construct as existing scales.

Floor and ceiling effects are quantified by calculating the proportion of study participants who score the minimum or maximum score. A floor or ceiling effect is considered to be present if $\geq 15\%$ of participants score the minimum or maximum score, respectively [1, 2]. If there is a floor or ceiling effect present, the scale needs to be recalibrated as it is measuring too high or low a level of that domain, respectively. For instance, if a scale measuring physical function demonstrates a floor effect (large proportion of patients scoring the minimum score), then the scale is "too hard" because it is calibrated to measure a level of physical function that is too difficult for the population being tested to achieve. Conversely, if a physical function scale demonstrates a ceiling effect, it is "too easy," and the population of interest has a higher level of physical function than the scale is calibrated to measure.

Translation and Cross-Cultural Adaptation

After a scale is developed, validated, and utilized, there is a frequent need to administer that scale in other countries and languages. Rather than simply translating a PROM word-for-word and implementing it in another language, there is an accepted methodology for performing scale translation and cross-cultural adaptation, which accounts for possible cultural differences between the initial scale language and the new translation.

Take, for instance, a scale developed in English that would be useful for a study being conducted in Japan. First, the scale is translated from English to Japanese by either a certified medical translator or an individual who is fluent in both languages and also understands the clinical construct being measured. Next, another individual back-translates the scale from Japanese into English. The investigators then compare the original English version to the back-translated English version to ensure the content has not changed. If they are concordant, then the Japanese (translated) version of the scale can move on to validation. If they are not concordant, the investigators must troubleshoot the reasons for the discrepancy and correct them. This ensures preservation of the meanings of the original questions.

The validation process can be done by one or both of the following methods:

1. Investigators can perform a full re-validation by comparing the translated scale to other validated scales in the target language measuring a similar construct.
2. Investigators can recruit research participants in the target demographic who are fluent in both languages. They can then administer one language version of the scale (e.g., the Japanese or English version, selected at random) at time one, followed by the other language version of the scale at time two (frequently 7 to 14 days later). Like reliability testing (Fig. 15.1), the translated scale is administered at time two with a "change" question to ensure that the participant has not had any relevant health status changes in the interval. By demonstrating reliability (with absolute agreement) with the scale in the original language, the new language adaptation is considered an acceptable reproduction of the original.

This chapter provided a broad overview of outcome scale development and validation techniques. Additional techniques including factor analysis and item response theory are beyond the scope of this text; further reading should include work by Robert DeVellis [3].

Analytical Review

> # Development and Validation of a Pediatric Sports Activity Rating Scale
>
> ## The Hospital for Special Surgery Pediatric Functional Activity Brief Scale (HSS Pedi-FABS)
>
> Peter D. Fabricant, MD, MPH, Alex Robles, BS, Timothy Downey-Zayas, BS, Huong T. Do, MA, Robert G. Marx, MD, MSc, Roger F. Widmann, MD, and Daniel W. Green, MD, MS

Fig. 15.2 Illustrative example of an outcome scale development and validation study by Fabricant et al. [4]

An example of a outcome scale development and validation study is illustrated in (Fig. 15.2).

As the field of pediatric orthopedic sports medicine was rapidly expanding in 2013, it became evident that there was no activity rating scale for children and adolescents. This was an important gap in the armamentarium of research instruments because it was impossible to quantify the amount of physical activity in children. This was despite the fact that the entire field of pediatric orthopedic sports medicine is focused on maintaining and increasing childhood activity levels after patients recover from orthopedic injuries. For adults, there was an existing activity rating scale designed for use after knee surgery, which quantified activity based on frequency alone [5]. Its use in children and adolescents was not appropriate because they participate in a wide range of physical activities of different intensity, and measurement based on activity frequency alone would be inadequate. For example, a child who performs running activities 5 days per week for 30 minutes only at mandatory physical education class would have been counted the same as a classmate who is going to the same physical education class and also running 5 times per week for 2 hours during varsity football practice. It became clear that additional domains to quantify the quality of activity, duration, and level of competition were necessary in order to appropriately stratify young patients.

The initial phase of the study involved item generation by a panel of orthopedic surgeons and adolescent athletes. Item reduction was performed by a separate cohort of 20 adolescent athletes to score the importance and frequency of each activity item, the total of which was then averaged. A concise 8-item questionnaire was created to minimize questionnaire fatigue. Pilot testing was then performed by 20 young athletes in clusters of five, who provided feedback regarding the language, layout, and ease of completion. After minor modifications, the scale was finalized when no further ambiguity remained (Fig. 15.3).

Instructions: Choose <u>one</u> answer for each activity or question. In the grid, please indicate how often you performed each activity in your healthiest and most active condition. IN THE PAST **MONTH**:

	Less than one time per month	One time per month	One time per week	2-3 times per week	More than 4 times per week
Running: running while playing a sport or jogging.					
Cutting: quickly changing directions while running.					
Decelerating: coming to a quick stop while running.					
Pivoting: turning your body with your foot planted (for example: skiing, skating, kicking, throwing, hitting a ball)					
Duration: perform athletic activity for as long as you would like to without stopping.					
Endurance: perform athletic activity for one whole hour without stopping.					

Competition: Do you participate in organized competitive sports or physical activities?

☐ No (or gym class only)

☐ Yes, but WITHOUT an official or judge (such as club or pickup games)

☐ Yes, WITH an official or judge

☐ Yes, at a national or professional level

Supervision: Do you participate in supervised (coach, trainer, instructor) sports practice or activities (other than gym class)?

☐ No

☐ Yes, 1-2 times per week

☐ Yes, 3-4 times per week

☐ Yes, 5 or more times per week

Fig. 15.3 The Hospital for Special Surgery Pediatric Functional Activity Brief Scale (HSS Pedi-FABS) [4]

To assess the validity of the scale, it was administered to 51 healthy, active adolescent participants 10 to 18 years old. Convergent validity was evaluated by comparing Hospital for Special Surgery Pediatric Functional Activity Brief Scale (HSS Pedi-FABS) scores to similar adult scales (Marx and Noyes), the Pediatric Activity Questionnaire (PAQ-A and PAQ-C), and participant-reported level of competition and weekly hours of sports participation. Discriminant validity was assessed by ensuring that the questionnaire responses did not differ significantly by participant age, body mass index, or Daniel scale (a 3-point scale that collects information about type of sport, but not frequency or intensity).

Test–retest reliability was assessed by asking the same participants to complete the questionnaire at an average of 7 days after the initial validation date and evaluating only those that also reported no change in their health in the interim (41 of the 51 participants). Internal consistency was calculated on all 51 participants' first questionnaire responses using Cronbach's alpha. Floor and ceiling effects were evaluated by the proportion of respondents who scored the lowest or highest possible scores, respectively.

The results showed statistically significant, moderate-strength correlations for the convergent validity analyses and no significant correlations for tests of discriminant validity. The scale demonstrated a high test–retest reliability (ICC = 0.91) and internal consistency (Cronbach's alpha = 0.91). There were no floor or ceiling effects, despite the presence of substantial ceiling effects when administering the adult scales to this population of pediatric and adolescent participants (4% with the maximum score on the new scale compared with 33%–57% reaching the maximum score on the adult scales). Therefore, it was concluded that the new activity scale is valid and reliable in measuring activity level in the pediatric and adolescent population.

Since its initial development and validation, this scale has been studied epidemiologically for baseline activity levels in American youth [6, 7], cross-validated to physical fitness testing [8] and other PROMs [9–12], and translated and culturally adapted into Japanese [13], Dutch [14], Italian [15], and French [16].

References

1. Terwee CB, Bot SD, de Boer MR, et al. Quality criteria were proposed for measurement properties of health status questionnaires. J Clin Epidemiol. 2007;60:34–42. https://doi.org/10.1016/j.jclinepi.2006.03.012.
2. McHorney CA, Tarlov AR. Individual-patient monitoring in clinical practice: are available health status surveys adequate? Qual Life Res Int J Qual Life Asp Treat Care Rehab. 1995;4:293–307. https://doi.org/10.1007/BF01593882.
3. DeVellis RF, Thorpe CT. Scale development: theory and applications. 5th ed. Thousand Oaks, CA: Sage Publications; 2021.
4. Fabricant PD, Robles A, Downey-Zayas T, et al. Development and validation of a pediatric sports activity rating scale: the Hospital for Special Surgery Pediatric Functional Activity Brief Scale (HSS Pedi-FABS). Am J Sports Med. 2013;41:2421–9. https://doi.org/10.1177/0363546513496548.
5. Marx RG, Stump TJ, Jones EC, et al. Development and evaluation of an activity rating scale for disorders of the knee. Am J Sports Med. 2001;29:213–8. https://doi.org/10.1177/0363546501029002160 1.
6. Fabricant PD, Suryavanshi JR, Calcei JG, et al. The Hospital for Special Surgery Pediatric Functional Activity Brief Scale (HSS Pedi-FABS): normative data. Am J Sports Med. 2018;46:1228–34. https://doi.org/10.1177/0363546518756349.
7. Fabricant PD, McLaren SH, Suryavanshi JR, et al. Association between government health insurance status and physical activity in American youth. J Pediatr Orthop. 2019;39:e552–7. https://doi.org/10.1097/BPO.0000000000001329.
8. Fabricant PD, Robles A, McLaren SH, et al. Hospital for Special Surgery Pediatric Functional Activity Brief Scale predicts physical fitness testing performance. Clin Orthop Relat Res. 2014;472:1610–6. https://doi.org/10.1007/s11999-013-3429-1.
9. Adjei J, Schachne JM, Green DW, et al. Correlation between the PROMIS pediatric mobility instrument and the Hospital for Special Surgery Pediatric Functional Activity Brief Scale (HSS Pedi-FABS). HSS J. 2020;16:311–5. https://doi.org/10.1007/s11420-019-09726-7.
10. Wagner KJ, Sabatino MJ, Zynda AJ, et al. Activity measures in pediatric athletes: a comparison of the Hospital for Special Surgery Pediatric Functional Activity Brief Scale and Tegner Activity Level Scale. Am J Sports Med. 2020;48:985–90. https://doi.org/10.1177/0363546520904009.

11. Iversen MD, von Heideken J, Farmer E, et al. Validity and comprehensibility of physical activity scales for children with sport injuries. J Pediatr Orthop. 2016;36:278–83. https://doi.org/10.1097/BPO.0000000000000448.

12. Yau A, Heath MR, Nguyen JT, et al. Legacy patient-reported outcome measures can be reliably translated to PROMIS domains for use in adolescent spinal deformity. Spine. 2021;46:e1254–61. https://doi.org/10.1097/BRS.0000000000004081.

13. Hozumi T, Akagi R, Fabricant PD, et al. Cross-cultural adaptation and validation of the Japanese version of the Hospital for Special Surgery Pediatric Functional Activity Brief Scale (HSS Pedi-FABS). Orthop J Sports Med. 2022;10:232596712211132. https://doi.org/10.1177/23259671221113284.

14. Dietvorst M, van de Kerkhof TM, Janssen RPA, et al. Translation and transcultural validation of the Dutch hospital for special surgery paediatric functional activity brief scale (HSS Pedi-FABS). BMC Musculoskelet Disord. 2021;22:853. https://doi.org/10.1186/s12891-021-04729-0.

15. Macchiarola L, Grassi A, Di Paolo S, et al. The Italian cross-cultural adaptations of the paediatric International Knee Documentation Committee Score and the Hospital for Special Surgery Paediatric Functional Activity Brief Scale are reliable instruments in paediatric population. Knee Surg Sports Traumatol Arthrosc. 2020;28:2657–62. https://doi.org/10.1007/s00167-020-05903-y.

16. Bel MJD, Kemp LG, Girard CI, et al. Translation and validation of the Hospital for Special Surgery Pediatric Functional Activity Brief Scale for French paediatric populations. Physiother Can. 2020;72:348–54. https://doi.org/10.3138/ptc-2019-0033.

Glossary

A priori Latin term meaning "from the earlier" or "from the cause"; used to describe research or decisions made before collecting data or conducting an experiment, respectively

Adaptive randomization A method of group assignment in randomized clinical trials where the probability of assigning a participant to a specific treatment group changes during the trial based on participant characteristics

Alpha (α) Alpha is the level of significance used in hypothesis testing, often set at 0.05, representing the probability of making a type I error. This is also known as the risk of making a false positive conclusion (rejecting the null hypothesis when there is in fact no difference between groups).

As-treated analysis An analysis method in clinical trials where participants are analyzed according to the treatment they actually received, rather than their randomized treatment assignment

Attrition bias A form of bias that occurs when participants drop out of a study, leading to a distorted representation of the population being studied

Bar chart A graphical representation of data using bars to display the frequency of categorical data

Beta (β) Beta represents the probability of making a type II error, which is failing to reject a false null hypothesis. This is also known as the risk of making a false negative conclusion.

Binary Refers to data or variables that have two distinct categories or values

Bivariable (or bivariate) statistics Both terms refer to the statistical analysis of the relationship between two variables in a dataset

Bonferroni correction A method used to adjust the significance level (alpha) when performing multiple comparisons to reduce the chance of a type I error

Boxplot A graphical representation of the distribution of data using median, quartiles, and outliers

© The Editor(s) (if applicable) and The Author(s), under exclusive license to Springer Nature Switzerland AG 2024
P. D. Fabricant, *Practical Clinical Research Design and Application*,
https://doi.org/10.1007/978-3-031-58380-3

Case-control study This is a study design where cases and controls are sampled based on the presence or absence of an outcome. Then patients are compared to see if they had previously experienced the exposure(s) of interest.

Categorical data Data structured as categories or groups and is often qualitative or nominal

Central tendency A statistical measure used to determine the center of a distribution (e.g., mean, median, mode)

Chi-squared test A statistical test used to determine whether there is a significant association between categorical variables

Clinical outcome scale A measurement tool used in healthcare to assess patient health status, symptoms, or quality of life

Cohort study An observational study where a group of individuals sharing a common characteristic are followed over time to observe outcomes

Comparative cohort study This is a study design where a cohort is classified based on experiencing an exposure (the independent variable). Then the cohort is queried on an outcome (the dependent variable).

Confounder, confounding variable A variable that influences both the independent variable and the dependent variable, which can distort the relationship between them and lead to a spurious association

Continuous data Data that can take any value within a range

Control group In an experiment, a group that does not receive the treatment being studied and is used as a comparison to assess the effects of the treatment

Convergent validity A type of validity that is demonstrated when a clinical outcome scale is associated with similar constructs or objective performance indicators to which it would be expected to be related

Correlation analysis Statistical analysis used to determine the relationship or association between two continuous variables

Covariable A variable that is statistically controlled for or adjusted in analyses due to its potential influence on the relationship between other variables

Covariance A measure of the relationship between two variables, indicating how much they change together

Crossover In a randomized clinical trial, a patient crossover refers to a situation where participants switch from one treatment or intervention to another during the course of the study

Crossover study design In a crossover trial, each participant receives multiple treatments in a specific sequence. This is the most rigorous study design within randomized trials because each study participant acts as his or her own internal control.

Cross-sectional study An observational study that collects data from a population at a single point in time

Cross-validation A technique used in model validation to assess how well a statistical model generalizes to an independent dataset

Data safety monitoring board (DSMB) A DSMB is an independent committee of experts established to oversee the safety and integrity of a clinical trial or study.

Its primary responsibility is to safeguard the interests of study participants, assess data quality, monitor safety parameters, and provide ongoing review and recommendations regarding the continuation, modification, or termination of a trial.

Descriptive statistics Statistical methods used to summarize and describe the basic features of a dataset

Directed acyclic graph (DAG) A graphical method to assist with study design which illustrates potential relationships and causal structures between variables

Discriminant validity A type of validity that is demonstrated when a clinical outcome scale is not associated with dissimilar constructs to which it should not be related

Double-blinded Refers to a study design where neither the participants nor the researchers are aware of who is receiving the treatment and who is in the control group

Effect modification (interaction) When the relationship between an exposure (independent variable) and an outcome (dependent variable) is different depending on the level or presence of another variable (effect modifier)

Effect size A measure used in statistical analysis to quantify the strength or magnitude of an observed effect

Equipoise "Clinical equipoise" refers to a state of uncertainty or disagreement among medical experts regarding the effectiveness of different available treatments.

Exchangeability Exchangeability is the measurement of comparability between treatment groups and is essential to causal inference between outcome and exposure. If two groups have identical characteristics except the exposure of interest, then they are considered to be "exchangeable".

Experimental study design A research design where the researcher actively manipulates one or more variables to observe the effect on another variable

Explanatory variable Independent or predictor variable

Exposure The factor or variable being studied to determine its effect on an outcome

False negative False negative is the failure to reject a false null hypothesis or the failure to detect a true effect or condition. See also: beta (β), Type II error

False positive False positive is the incorrect rejection of a true null hypothesis or a false detection of an effect or condition that is not actually present. See also: alpha (α), Type I error

Financial bias Bias that arises due to financial interests influencing research outcomes or decisions

Floor and ceiling effects When data cluster at the lower or upper extremes of a measurement scale, limiting the ability to discern differences among patients or research participants

Histogram A graphical representation of the distribution of numerical data using bars to display frequency

Hypothesis testing A statistical method used to make inferences about a population based on sample data

Incidence The rate of occurrence of new cases of a disease or condition within a specified period of time

Independent predictor A variable that predicts the outcome variable while controlling for other variables in a statistical model

Independent samples *t*-test A statistical test used to compare means between two independent groups

Information bias Bias caused by errors or inaccuracies in the collection, interpretation, or recording of data

Incorporation bias Incorporation bias is bias that occurs when the results of a test or variable in question is part of (or incorporated into) the reference test (or gold standard). Bias occurs because the outcome is directly due in part to incorporation of the predictor variable in determining the outcome.

Intention-to-treat analysis An analysis that includes all participants according to their original assigned groups, regardless of protocol deviations or non-compliance

Interaction See effect modification

Interquartile range (IQR) A measure of statistical dispersion representing the range between the first and third quartiles in a dataset

Interrater reliability A measurement of the extent to which multiple data collectors or assessors (raters) assign the same score to the same variable or measurement

Intraclass correlation coefficient (ICC) A measure used to assess reliability or agreement among different observers or raters

Intrarater reliability The consistency or stability of measurements made by the same rater on multiple occasions

Item reduction A process in scale development where duplicate or similar items are eliminated to create a more concise and efficient scale

Kappa A statistic used to measure inter-rater agreement or reliability for categorical items, correcting for chance agreement

Kurtosis Kurtosis is a statistical measure used to describe the shape, or peakedness, of the probability distribution of a dataset. It assesses the degree to which the distribution deviates from a normal distribution in terms of the tails and the central peak.

Linear regression A statistical method used to model the relationship between a continuous outcome variable and one or more predictor variables

Logistic regression A statistical technique used to model the relationship between a binary outcome variable and one or more predictor variables

Main effect In statistics, the effect of a single independent variable on a dependent variable without considering other variables

McNemar test A statistical test used to determine if there is a significant change in proportions or frequencies between paired observations; also known as a paired or matched samples chi-squared test

Mean Also known as the average, the mean is calculated by adding up all the values in a dataset and dividing the sum by the total number of values. It is sensitive to extreme values (outliers) and is affected by their presence in the dataset.

Median The median is the middle value in a dataset when the values are arranged in ascending or descending order. If the dataset has an odd number of values, the median is the middle number. If the dataset has an even number of values, the median is the average of the two middle numbers. The median is less affected by extreme values.

Mediator A variable that explains or acts as a link in the relationship between an independent variable and a dependent variable

Misclassification Misclassification refers to the incorrect categorization or labeling of data points or individuals in a dataset. It can be differential (e.g., systematically varied between groups) or nondifferential (e.g., similar for all groups), and can result in incorrect study conclusions.

Mode The value that occurs most frequently in a dataset, and can be used with numerical and categorical data

Multivariable statistics See regression analysis, linear regression, and logistic regression

Negative predictive value The probability that a negative test result is a true negative

Nonparametric analysis Statistical methods used when the assumptions of parametric statistics are not met, for instance when dealing with non-normally distributed data

Null hypothesis The null hypothesis is a statement that suggests there is no effect or no difference between groups and conditions in a study. Rejection of a null hypothesis indicates that there is an effect or difference between groups.

Observational study design A research design where the researcher observes and collects data without intervening or manipulating variables

Observer bias Bias that occurs due to the behavior or expectations of the researcher or observer

Odds ratio A measure of association used in case-control studies to estimate the odds of exposure in cases compared to controls

Operationalization The process of defining abstract concepts though measurable observations, and quantifiably defining variables to make them useful for clinical research

Outlier data Outlier data refers to observations or data points that significantly differ from the majority of the other data points in a dataset. These points lie exceptionally far from the bulk of the data and may not follow the same pattern or distribution as the rest of the dataset.

Parametric data Data that follows a normal distribution and therefore meets the assumptions of parametric statistics

Patient-reported outcome measures (PROMs) Instruments used to assess a patient's health status or experience which are directly reported by the patient

Phase I trial The initial stage of clinical trials assessing the safety and tolerability of a new treatment in a small group of (typically healthy) participants

Phase II trial The second stage of clinical trials evaluating the efficacy and safety of a new treatment in a larger group of participants (typically affected with the disease being studied)

Phase III trial These trials are large-scale clinical trials comparing the new treatment to standard treatment to determine its effectiveness, safety, and side effects. This is typically a randomized controlled trial or crossover study.

Phase IV trial Post-marketing surveillance conducted after a drug or treatment is approved to monitor its safety and effectiveness in a larger population

Placebo effect A beneficial effect on a person's condition resulting from a placebo treatment, often due to psychological factors

Placebo treatment A harmless substance or inactive treatment given to participants in the control group during a clinical trial

Positive predictive value The probability that a positive test result is a true positive

Power calculation A statistical computation used to determine the sample size required to detect a specific effect size or difference between groups

Prevalence The proportion of a population with a particular disease or condition at a specific point in time

Propensity score A score used to match or adjust for a set of potential confounding variables in observational studies

Prospective cohort study An observational study where participants are enrolled and followed over time to observe outcomes based on exposure

Publication bias Publication bias occurs when the publication of research findings is influenced by the nature or direction of the results, rather than the rigor of the study. Published studies are more likely to report statistically significant results than negative findings.

R^2 value (coefficient of determination) A measure in regression analysis representing the proportion of variability in the dependent variable explained by the independent variable(s) included in a regression model

Random error Variation in data caused by chance or inherent variability, which can be minimized by increasing sample size or improving measurement techniques

Randomization Randomization is the process of assigning participants to different groups in a study by chance to reduce bias and ensure equal representation of all covariables. This allows the intervention to be the only difference between the groups.

Randomized controlled trial (RCT) RCT is an experimental study design which is considered the gold standard for assessing the safety and efficacy of medical interventions. They allow researchers to establish causal relationships between interventions and outcomes.

Rate ratio The rate ratio is calculated as the ratio of the incidence rates (or rates of occurrence) of an outcome in two distinct groups and helps quantify the strength and direction of the association between exposure and outcome. It cannot be used in case-control study designs because it depends on the frequency of an outcome which in a case-control study design is preset by the investigator.

Receiver operating characteristic (ROC) curve A graphical plot used to evaluate the performance of a diagnostic test by plotting sensitivity against 1 minus the specificity

Recall bias A type of bias caused by differences in the accuracy or completeness of participant recall or memory of an exposure or outcome

Regression analysis A statistical method used to examine the relationship between a dependent variable and one or more independent variables

Relative risk The ratio of the risk of an event in one group compared to another group

Reporting bias Bias that occurs when the results or outcomes of a study are selectively reported, influencing the perception of the findings

Retrospective cohort study (or case series) A type of observational study that uses historical patient data or records in order to evaluate outcomes based on prior exposure

Risk ratio The ratio of the probability of an event occurring in an exposed group compared to an unexposed group

ROC curve See Receiver Operating Characteristic curve

Sample size The number of individuals or units included in a study or analysis, which affects the power, precision, and generalizability of the results

Sensitivity The measure of a test's ability to correctly identify as many disease-positive patients as possible and is calculated as the proportion of patients who have the disease who test positive

Selection bias A bias that occurs when the selection of patients or study participants is not random, leading to a non-representative sample

Simple randomization A method of randomizing participants to different groups where each participant has an equal chance of being assigned to any group

Significance level See alpha (α)

Skewness Skewness is a statistical measure that describes the asymmetry or lack of symmetry in the distribution of a dataset. It measures the degree and direction of deviation from a symmetric, normal distribution.

Specificity The measure of a test's ability to correctly identify as many disease-negative patients as possible and is calculated as the proportion of patients without the disease who test negative

Standard deviation A measure of the dispersion or spread of data points around the mean in a dataset

Statistical bias Systematic error or deviation from the true value caused by flaws in the study design, analysis, or interpretation

Statistical power The probability that a study will detect an effect or difference when one truly exists ($1 - $ type II error rate $[\beta]$)

Threshold value In diagnostic testing, the cutoff point used to determine a positive or negative result based on test values

True negative In diagnostic testing, a correct negative test result indicating the absence of a condition in an individual without the condition

True positive In diagnostic testing, a correct positive test result indicating the presence of a condition in an individual with the condition

Type I error See false positive, alpha (α)

Type II error See false negative, beta (β)

Univariable statistics Statistical analysis involving one variable at a time, often used to describe or analyze individual variables independently

Validity The extent to which a measurement or test accurately measures what it is intended to measure

Youden index A statistic used in diagnostic testing to identify the optimal cutoff point for a diagnostic test, balancing sensitivity and specificity

z-test A statistical test that is used to determine whether there is a significant difference between the means of two large independent samples, or between the mean of a sample and that of a known population when the population standard deviation is known

Index

P. D. Fabricant, *Practical Clinical Research Design and Application*,
https://doi.org/10.1007/978-3-031-58380-3

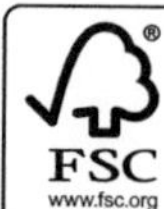